WHAT TO
DO WHEN
THE DOCTOR
SAYS IT'S

ENDOMETRIOSIS

WHAT TO DO WHEN THE DOCTOR SAYS IT'S

ENDOMETRIOSIS

Everything You Need to Know to Stop the Pain
and Heal Your Fertility

THOMAS LYONS, M.D.
and CHERYL KIMBALL

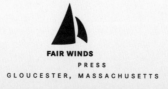

FAIR WINDS
PRESS
GLOUCESTER, MASSACHUSETTS

Text © 2003 by Cheryl Kimball & Thomas Lyons, M.D.

First published in the USA in 2003 by
Fair Winds Press
33 Commercial Street
Gloucester, MA 01930

Library of Congress Cataloging-in-Publication Data

Kimball, Cheryl.
What to do when the doctor says it's endometriosis : everything you need to know to stop the pain and heal your fertility / Cheryl Kimball and Thomas Lyons.
    p. cm.
Includes bibliographical references and index.
ISBN 1-59233-029-0
1. Endometriosis--Popular works. I. Lyons, Thomas (Thomas L.) II. Title.
RG483.E53K54 2003
618.1--dc22
                              2003018250

ISBN 1-59233-029-0

10 9 8 7 6 5 4 3 2 1

Cover design by Laura Shaw Design
Book design by Susan Raymond

Printed and bound in Canada

The information in this book is for educational purposes only. It is not intended to replace the advice of a physician or medical practitioner.

We dedicate this book to the many thousands of women who suffer with endometriosis and their families who have suffered with them.

We wish to thank the people who have helped us write the book, both the patients who have shared their stories and the mentors who taught us how to take care of the patient not just the disease.

Personally, I would like to thank my family, who put up with me while I labor in my obsessions.

—Tom Lyons

There are always many people to thank when it comes to writing a book:

First and foremost, I would like to thank Dr. Lyons for enthusiastically jumping on board with this project. My experience working with him reinforces the glowing praise he received from the women I interviewed who have been his patients. He is clearly a kind, compassionate, and thoroughly dedicated doctor. And to top it off, he's got a great sense of humor!

Not far behind is my appreciation to Sue Ducharme, who helped with the research and writing of several chapters. This is a woman who knows the value of deadlines. No wonder she is in demand as a freelance editor.

Patrice Dickey, PD Communications, works with Dr. Lyons on PR and publicity and was an enthusiastic and helpful source of interview candidates. Many thanks go to her.

And thanks go to those women who let me pry into their medical history and get them to relive some painful experiences. They all are determined to let their experiences help other women and I appreciate their time.

—Cheryl Kimball

CONTENTS

CHAPTER ONE ౿

What Is Endometriosis?
What Causes It and What Does It Do to My Body?

For women with endometriosis, the answer to "what is it?" is simple: Endometriosis is what's keeping you from living your life to the fullest. Because endometriosis causes pain, as well as other symptoms, this problem keeps some women in bed for several days each month. Other women have chronic low-level pain that just hangs on day after day after day with little relief. And some have menstrual flow so heavy that they can't stray too far from a bathroom and a supply of feminine products.

You can't plan a weekend away because you just don't know if you will be up for the trip. Since your teenage years, you were the family "sick kid." No reunion, family picnic, or holiday gathering went by without you either feeling too ill to attend or ending up curled up in your aunt's bedroom unable to participate in the fun.

Endometriosis impacts a woman's ability to develop a relationship or to maintain an intimate relationship. Sex is often painful. And to top it off, endometriosis often compromises fertility, making it difficult to conceive.

Does this sound familiar?

Despite the fact that endometriosis affects approximately six million women in the United States alone, very few people understand the disease or how much it can change a woman's life. Other people can't see anything wrong with you, which makes it hard for them to figure out why you miss work unexpectedly several days a month. Or why you simply don't feel like going to the mall or the movies. Not everyone can understand that just chatting over a cup of coffee seems like too much to deal with for someone in pain.

If these problems sound like yours, this book will show you how to seize the day and develop a whole new attitude. After years of practice and helping women with endometriosis, I know that you and your doctors can turn the tide, so that endometriosis does not control you, you control it.

Now let's get through the technical details about what endometriosis actually is and what it does to your body to cause you pain and suffering. Then we can get on to the good stuff: The information that will tell you how to move endometriosis out of the limelight of your life.

The Technical Stuff

Endometrium is the name of the tissue that lines the uterus. This lining thickens on a cyclical basis in anticipation of accommodating a growing fetus. When sperm and egg do not arrive to settle into this soft nest, the lining sheds in the form of the menstrual period and the body recreates the lining in a few weeks.

Endometriosis, according to the Merriam-Webster Dictionary, is "the presence of functioning endometrial tissue in places where it does not belong."

In approximately 10 percent of adult pre-menopausal women, endometrial tissue appears outside of the uterus. However, even though the tissue is not in the uterus, it still reacts to the hormonal stimulation that causes the monthly menstrual cycle. So this misplaced tissue attempts to go through the same process as healthy endometrial tissue. It engorges with blood and then attempts to shed blood and tissue when conception does not occur. In other words, even though the tissue isn't in your uterus, it acts as if it is, growing and changing as time goes by.

The key difference between the healthy endometrial lining and the misplaced tissue is that the healthy tissue is able to exit the body each month through menstruation but the errant endometrial tissue has nowhere to go. We think the attempted shedding of tissue and blood may be one cause of the high level of pain associated with endometriosis.

Likewise, the unshed blood and tissue cause adhesions, lumps, and lesions, which are in themselves painful. The pain caused by this tissue and its growth and potential shedding is so dramatic and intense (unlike, say, traditional menstrual cramps), that it is impossible to ignore or relieve with over-the-counter pain medications.

We do not know what causes endometriosis nor do we have a sure-fire cure. However, women with endometriosis have many options that can alleviate their pain in the future.

Pardon the Slang

Endometriosis is a long word, and to make this book a little less cumbersome I occasionally used the shortened term "endo." Although this is a commonly accepted and well-used abbreviation, I want to assure you that I am in no way trying to put a casual slant on this complex and often debilitating condition by using the shortened term. I use endo as opposed to the full word merely for ease of reading; and I only use the shortened version when the word endometriosis comes up several times in succession, which happens more than occasionally.

A Few Definitions

The glossary in the back of this book has definitions of words that come up a lot when you're dealing with endo. However, here are a few words that are helpful to understand up front.

Endometrium: As mentioned above, endometrium is the medical term for the lining of the uterus. The word is Latin and breaks down to *endo*, meaning "inside," and *metrium*, meaning "mother."

Implants, lesions, nodules: Doctors use all three of these terms to describe areas of endometrial tissue found in parts of the body outside of the uterus.

Endocrinologist: This is the medical specialist who focuses on the hormone-producing system of the body known as the endocrine system. Medical endocrinologists treat diabetes, thyroid disorders, and other hormonal imbalances. Reproductive endocrinologists (REs) are gynecologists who treat disorders of the female hormone system. REs are the doctors who treat disorders of the female hormone system and infertility.

Too Common
Endometriosis affects approximately six million women in America—between eight and 10 percent of women of reproductive age—making it one of the most common gynecological dieases.

Of this number, 30 to 40 percent of affected women are infertile, making endometriosis appear to be one of the leading causes of infertility in women. This statistic, however, may actually be more of a case of guilt by association, rather than a true case of cause and effect. The research is still out on this, but the good news is that we often treat infertility associated with endo very successfully with hormone therapy, surgery, or both. In fact, during pregnancy the symptoms of endometriosis seem to subside, sometimes significantly. Unfortunately, the disease does not go away and symptoms will likely recur after a woman has finished her pregnancy and breast feeding.

Sometimes doctors encourage women with endometriosis to rush into getting pregnant, but there is no well-researched medical rationale for this recommendation. I discuss all of the fertility issues involving endometriosis, including some potential complications, in Chapter Nine.

How Does It Happen?

Even though we live in an era of advanced medical research and knowledge, we still don't understand how endometrial tissue ends up outside the uterus. There are several theories, but none are definitive. Perhaps all of the theories are right, with each patient experiencing a different path to this condition. The possibilities include the following:

- The uterine lining, the endometrium, may expand up through the fallopian tubes into the abdomen, where it implants and grows. We presume that this happens because of an immune system or hormone problem, making the implantation of the endometrium actually a symptom of an underlying hormonal or immune condition. In other words, a woman may have another problem, but the most prominent symptom is pelvic pain, which leads the doctor to consider endometriosis as a diagnosis. I have included information on some of these hormonal and immune system problems in the book, in case you are a patient who suspects this situation is true of you.

- Perhaps menstrual blood, instead of draining out of the body, backs up through the fallopian tubes into the pelvic cavity, where it attaches to whatever surface it meets. This theory presumes a girl who has not yet started her menstrual cycle cannot suffer from endometrisis.

- The vascular theory states that endometrial tissue begins to travel through the blood or through the lymph system.

- The congenital theory states that in the embryo, cells that are intended to form the uterus don't arrive before the uterus has closed in development. These cells are present outside the uterus at birth, which means that some women may be born with endometriosis.

- The metaplasia theory states that cells develop abnormally and in locations where they don't belong. Again, these cells would be present when you are born.

Endometriosis is most often found in the pelvic area, with tissue attaching just outside the uterus, around the ovaries, and on the fallopian tubes. Lesions are also commonly found in the abdominal cavity, including near the intestines, colon, and bladder. Less common are endo lesions in distant parts of the body, such as behind the knees or near the lungs. This is, yet again, another reason why pelvic pain is most often the first known symptom of endometriosis.

The Dioxin Connection

Why endometriosis happens is even more of a mystery than how it actually occurs. If you do any research on endometriosis (and you should!), you will find a lot of discussion and research on the effects of the chemical compound dioxin. Dioxin is one of the most toxic synthetic chemicals in existence. When herbicides, such as the infamous Agent Orange used in the Vietnam War, break down, dioxin is what's left. "Dioxin is an environmental toxicant that alters the action of estrogen in reproductive organs and adversely affects immuno-competence," acccording to the National Institutes of Health. "Immuno-competence" is the ability of the immune system to function normally.

Researchers also suspect other chemical-related causes of endometriosis. Women in the second half of the 20th century commonly took a drug called diethylstilbestrol (DES) to prevent miscarriage. Many children of the women who took drug reached childbearing age and found they had fertility problems. Perhaps this medication and others like it, as well as chemical toxins, contribute to endometriosis.

Unfortunately, we still don't know the answer. The connection between toxins and endometriosis is certainly not definite. Howevever, we do know that our "miracle" chemicals and synthetic materials—think of DDT and asbestos—often have devastating long-term effects that aren't apparent in the first generation of use.

Because we aren't sure if or how much dioxin, DES, and other toxins are part of the endometriosis equation, I always suggest that women with endo eat a healthy organic diet, avoiding chemicals and hormones as much as possible. For more details, see Chapter Eight.

Related Diseases

Fortunately, we now know—definitively—that endometriosis is directly related to the health and function of the immune system. Many immune disorders, such as allergies, fibromyalgia, chronic fatigue syndrome, and skin problems such as eczema, coincide with endometriosis. This doesn't mean that endo causes these conditions or vice versa; instead we think they are somehow related.

So, even if you have symptoms that you don't think are connected to endometriosis, by all means bring them up with your doctor. For example, if you have both pelvic pain and bad allergies, tell your physician, rather than keeping silent about what seem to be unrelated symptoms. I have found that some of my patients feel like it's too difficult to deal with more than one thing at a time; but, in the end, you could feel worse physically, because another medical condition may contribute to, or at least be related to, your endometriosis symptoms.

In addition to related diseases, endometriosis symptoms can actually mimic the symptoms of other illness, too. For instance, pelvic inflammatory disease (PID), is a common example. Known for causing severe pain, PID is actually a sexually transmitted disease caused by the bacteria Chlamydia. The bacterial infection often causes urethritis, an inflammation of the urethra causing pain, burning, and discharge, and it can lead to infertility.

It's important to look at all of your symptoms, because endometriosis can only be definitively diagnosed through laparoscopic surgery. So, you and your physician will want to eliminate other potential conditions with symptoms similar to endo before you have to consider surgery.

I also recommend taking care of other symptoms and illnesses because the better your overall health, the easier you will be able to deal with the pain of endometriosis. If your body doesn't also have to cope with other symptoms that drag you down—allergies, for instance—then it will be better able to cope with your endo symptoms.

You will learn more about related health conditions that women with endometriosis might experience in Chapter Six.

Connection to Cancer?

Here is some very good news: Although anything is possible, even the most errant endometrial tissue is rarely cancerous. Nor does endometriosis signal any connection to other types of cancer. According to the Mayo Clinic Website, "having endometriosis does not increase a woman's risk of uterine or ovarian cancer." The National Institutes of Health concurs and indicates that less than 1 percent of endometriosis cases coincide with a form of cancer—a small statistic that would probably be similar for almost any chronic condition.

Diagnosis

One of the saddest aspects of endometriosis is how long it takes the average woman to get an actual diagnosis. I've had patients who struggled for as long as nine years before getting proper treatment. Fortunately, as endo becomes better understood and women become more proactive in leading their own health care team, this length of time should decrease.

If you tell your doctor about any type of pain and his response is, "It's normal," I suggest you find another physician. This is not an answer! Although sometimes the cause of pain is evident or accept-able (for example, if you hit your toe on a chair and it hurts afterward), pain of any kind is not a normal function of the body.

Even menstrual pain is not necessarily "normal." Women have been conditioned to accept their "lot in life" to "suffer through" their monthly cycle and just accept pain with menstruation. Don't fall for this! If you are experiencing pain—anything more than mild discomfort—every month, talk with your primary care physician and/or your gynecologist.

If your doctor dismisses your pain as "normal" or "in your head," consider going to see a more sympathetic physician (yes, there are some out there!). Although even doctors sometimes find pain hard to relate to since it can't be seen, they should take your perception seriously. A physician should never dismiss your feelings, thoughts, or ideas as unimportant. I explain more about approaches for work-ing with your doctor in Chapter 10 .

Another reason for the long delay in diagnosis is because of endo-metriosis' close relationship with infertility. Physicians sometimes don't take women seriously when they complain of pain, but do begin to listen to them once the woman explains that she can't get pregnant. If you have symptoms that you think may be part of endometriosis, don't give up on getting a diagnosis and definitely don't wait until you want to get pregnant before you receieve serious treatment. And even if you don't want to have a child, or have already had your children, take your symptoms seriously.

Constructing a Health Care Team

Along with some tips on how to work most effectively with your doctor, I discuss in Chapter Ten how important it is for you to organize a health care team, comprised of specialists who are on your side. First and foremost, you are the manager of the team. Only you can decide which doctors and specialists you are comfortable with and whose approach meets your own. You do the hiring—and firing. You weigh all the factors given to you by your team, you do your own research, and then you are the one to make the final decisions about your care.

Symptom Log

With most chronic conditions and definitely with endometriosis, you can help pinpoint a diagnosis by documenting your symptoms, including (and perhaps especially) pain. Buy a blank book and make it your personal health journal. Log all of your symptoms, whether or not you think they relate to endometriosis.

Don't dismiss anything as inconsequential. Keep track of your menstrual cycles—timing, duration, and flow. Unless you are too self-conscious to write it down, keep track of sexual intercourse and any pain you experience with it. Severe pain during and after inter-course is a common complaint of women with endometriosis, so women should keep track of the problem and do the best they can to tell their doctors about this symptom.

However, don't expect your doctor to read every word of your journal (and the fact that he/she won't, might make you less self-conscious about what you write!). Use the information in your journal to find common factors and patterns to tell your doctor, giving him/her a brief synopsis of your findings.

Seeing your symptoms on paper might help you, too, notice patterns that previously didn't occur to you. This is exactly the type of information that you should tell your doctor.

Questions to Ask Yourself

You will only know—definitively—if you have endometriosis if you have surgery, because that is the only way a physician can visually see and diagnose lesions. Nevertheless, because of the list of symptoms and your careful collection of research, you and your doctor will, at some point, be pretty sure that you have endometriosis. At this point, both you and your doctor will need to consider some issues, such as:

- *What is the most troubling aspect of endometriosis for you?* Fertility is a key concern for many women, but perhaps that isn't a concern for you at this stage of your life. Perhaps you are more concerned about the fact that you can't travel for your career because you never know when your endometriosis symptoms will debilitate you. Perhaps you are in a promising new relationship but because sexual intercourse is so painful, you feel scared to be intimate. Whatever you're most concerned about is OK—it is your life and your concerns may be different than those of others. You don't have to follow any sort of disease "norm."

- *How far are you willing to go in treatment?* Your answer to this will depend a lot on how severe your symptoms are. It may not even depend on how pervasive your endometriosis is, since some women have endo in many places in their bodies but do not have severe pain. Again, only you can decide the answer to this. Surgery, hormone treatments, alternative treatments, and other possibilities all come into play. This is where you need to do your homework to know just what factors are involved with each option.

Treatments
Surgery

Once you and your doctor suspect endometriosis, you may decide to have surgery, because a physician can only definitely diagnosis endometriosis if he or she actually sees the tissue outside of the uterus. Fortunately, a surgeon can also remove some or all of the endometrial lesions at the same time.

Surgeons usually perform this procedure with a laparoscope. First, the physicians distend your abdomen with a harmless gas to provide viewing room around your organs. Then, he makes tiny incisions through which he inserts a tiny camera and surgical instruments. The doctor watches a television-like monitor that shows the images from the camera to see what is going on inside your body.

Hormones

Many physicians recomend hormone treatments for endometriosis. Each type of treatment takes a little different attack on symptoms. For example, if your pain symptoms typically intensify right before your period, you can take birth control pills to regulate the normal cyclical growth of the endometrium, therefore reducing flow during menstruation and ultimately easing the pain.

Some hormones reduce or even stop your period, which can potentially reduce endometriosis and its sypmtoms for months and even years after you actually stop taking the medication.

All hormone treatments come with the potential for serious side effects, so you and your physician, whether he or she is a OB/GYN or an endocrinologist, need to carefully monitor your reaction to the medication.

The side effects can include acne, weight gain, and breast changes (such as tenderness). And, of course, there has been some evidence of increased cancer risks associated with hormone therapies.

If you do take hormones at any point during your endometriosis treatment, never stop taking a hormone "cold turkey." Always work with your doctor in stopping hormone treatments per her recommendation. Some hormone therapies (such as birth control pills) have a contraceptive effect. With other hormone treatments, you could still get pregnant but should use contraception while taking them, because some hormones (such as danocrine) can have harmful effects on an unborn child. Again, it is important to work with your doctor to be sure you are taking hormones in a safe and effective manner.

I devoted Chapter Three to the topic of medical (i.e., drugs opposed to surgery) treatment for endometriosis.

Alternative Approaches

More and more, my patients ask me about what they commonly call "alternative" or "complementary" approaches to treating endometriosis, as well as other problems. These approaches include acupuncture, herbal therapies, massage, and other treatments that Western physicians don't study in medical training.

Alternative approaches often especially help pain management, an important element of endometriosis care. As with anything related to your health, be sure to let your primary care doctor know which alternative treatments you want to consider or currently use, so that he can be keep them in mind when they are recommending and exploring your treatment program.

Chapter Seven outlines the various complementary options and their specific use in treating endometriosis.

Endometriosis and Menopause

Because hormones play a role in endometriosis, menopause (during which the hormone levels in women change drastically) can signal a vast reduction in endometriosis symptoms, but this is not always the case. Symptoms of this endometriosis may remain long after the cessation of natural hormonal activity during menopause.

Cure

The bottom line is that at this stage in our knowledge of endometriosis, surgical options are the closest we can come to a cure. As a surgeon, I have seen the significant changes that surgery for endometriosis has made on women's lives. I'll cover surgery in Chapter Six, but let me say early on that the surgery used today to help endometriosis patients is as noninvasive as surgery can possibly get. Done with small incisions and tiny cameras, the surgical treatment of endo is an incredible pain reliever and infertility cure. Eighty-five percent of women who have conservative but aggressive surgery to remove their endometriosis report considerable reduction of painful symptoms. Afterwards, coping with endo becomes a matter of managing the comparatively small amount of pain that sometimes remains.

The old adage that the cure for endometriosis is a hysterectomy with removal of the ovaries could not be further from the truth. Sometimes a hysterectomy is necessary, if there are problems with the uterus (such as bleeding, fibroid tumors, or pelvic prolapse), but it should not be considered a primary treatment for endo or related symptoms. Most women with endometriosis can have children, but they may have to make decisions faster or in a different time frame than if they didn't have endometriosis. If a doctor tells you that you need a hysterectomy and/or you will not be able to have children because of your endometriosis, be sure to get a second opinion.

And let me also say that surgery is not your only option. Even if you do choose surgery, it is not the only endometriosis treatment you will use to combat the disease.

Personal Stories

When we're going through a crisis in our lives or have a problem, it's helpful to know that someone else has successfully come through the other side of dealing with the same issue. Knowing that others understand how frustrated and angry you feel about dealing with pain every day of your life is very reassuring. At the end of several chapters in this book, women who have endometriosis will share their personal stories. These women will tell you the irritations they dealt with before getting a diagnosis, how they finally got one, and finally, their keys to gaining control of their disease and managing the symptoms. I hope that these stories will provide you with a "one-way support network."

The stories that the women in this book share may also bring up some new aspect of endometriosis and its management that you hadn't thought of or heard about. The stories cover surgical intervention (both hysterectomy, in the case of a woman who had completed her family, and "simple" laparoscopy, in the case of a younger women who suffered debilitating pain), drug therapy, and alternative therapies in combination with conventional treatments.

Read these stories with your own experience in mind. Understand that just because one woman had a hysterectomy does not mean that you will need or should have a hysterectomy. But these stories can provide you with an understanding of all the options when it comes to understanding and controlling a complex disease like endometriosis.

While these stories remain anonymous, first-name only (and sometimes that has been changed), the women interviewed were all enthusiastic about contributing. When told that the stories would keep their identity unknown, they all said something like, "You can print my complete name, first, middle, and last if you want. I am just happy if one other woman gets some help from my story."

As you might expect, not one of women in these stories underestimated what you may be going through. They've been there, they are still there, and they are generous with their time and experience.

The Future

The research community—medical schools, hospitals, drug companies, and other medical specialists—is very much interested in finding both a cause and a cure for endometriosis. Studies and clinical trials go on all the time for endo, including the possibility of finding a way to diagnose endometriosis through a blood test. If researchers could find a way to do this, it would eliminate the need for laparoscopic exploratory surgery as the only definitive diagnosis for endometriosis. Currently, however, the ability to diagnose endometriosis through a blood test isn't possible.

Participating in a clinical trial is not for everyone, but if you have a "help others" attitude and tend to heavily research your own health issues, it may interest you quite a bit. The Federal Government and the medical community carefully regulate clinical trials. Before you sign up, the researchers will explain every detail about the study up front, including whether it would put you in even the smallest amount of danger.

You can find out about upcoming clinical trials in a number of ways. First, check out some web sites that keep updated lists and give detailed information about trials, as well as offering information about what type participants they need to find:

- National Institutes of Health (NIH): These government-funded health research institutes provide a clinical trials Website (www.clinicaltrials.gov) that identifies health-related research studies. One interesting thing about this site is that you can even find information (such as the results of the study) about clinical trials that are no longer recruiting for participants.

As I write this, the NIH site listed three studies; two were with the National Institute of Child and Human Development in Bethesda, Maryland, and one was with the Oregon College of Oriental

Medicine (see Chapter Seven for more information on this upcoming study).

- CenterWatch: You can search the CenterWatch Website (www.centerwatch.com) by medical condition. When I looked up endometriosis, for example, I received a list of thirty-nine clinical trials taking place nationwide, including studies in Utah, Ohio, Florida, and Connecticut. CenterWatch also has a patient notification service that will keep you posted on up to twenty conditions you select, so you can let the organization know that you are interested in participating in an endometriosis study. CenterWatch keeps all the information you give to the organization completely confidential.

One of the trials listed on CenterWatch required the participants to live in the local area, but most of the thirty-eight other listings for endometriosis were for one national trial investigating a new pain drug. This is a typical description of the participants studies look for: pre-menopausal, between ages 18 and 45, in general good health, and not pregnant or breastfeeding, and must experience pelvic pain that has been diagnosed as endometriosis.

If you are interested in clinical trial—whether as a potential participant or just to find out about each study and its results—keep these two sites on your internet server's favorites list and check them once in a while. Another bonus for checking in with the sites on a regular basis: You can go to your next doctor's appointment with up-to-date information.

Both CenterWatch and NIH outline the specifics of how to get involved in a clinical trial. Here are some questions to ask if you want to get involved:

- Who is the sponsor of the trial? Often this will be a large pharmaceutical company or the NIH or some other government organization. You don't need to be overly suspicious if the trial is being sponsored by a drug company— they are under extremely tight regulations and scrutiny by federal agencies.

- Are there any costs to me for the trial? If you have to travel to the trial site and stay in a hotel for the duration, who is responsible for the costs? If you have to travel quite a distance every day for the trial, who pays for that commuting cost?

- Exactly what treatments are going to be used? Drugs, alternative therapies? Will there be x-rays involved? How will the drugs be administered?

The researchers will provide you with lots of literature and information on their study. You should very carefully read "the informed consent form." As the title implies, this lengthy piece of legalese will describe the study, what the patient can expect to have happen to her during the study, and any risks that may be involved with participating in the study, such as drug side effects.

Keep in mind that it is within your rights to opt out of a clinical trial at any time during the process, so if you find that the side effects or even just the necessary details of the study are too much for you, you don't have to stick it through to the end (although, of course, the researchers are counting on you to stay the course).

You should also plan to discuss your participation with your medical team. Have your doctor review the information about the study and explain if she has any questions or concerns. If she does, the researchers should be able to provide answers that satisfy both you and your doctor. Clinical trials have a contact person, such as a research assistant, to handle your questions. Once you understand the details of the study, you need to sign the informed consent form, which states that you have been fully informed and are signing your approval to participate.

Besides general research through clinical trials, drug companies always research new drugs for extended periods before they are put on the market. Likewise, they also research new uses for existing medications, which is how, for example, a drug can be approved to treat two separate ailments.

The U.S. Food and Drug Administration (FDA) approves all medications only for specific uses, so any new use must go through a rigorous approval process before the pharmaceutical company can promote the drug for a different illness than it was first created to alleviate. The good thing about new uses for existing drugs is that a lot is already known about potential side effects on humans. New drugs will have had years of testing on lab animals, but what a drug does to a mouse is not necessarily what it will do to a human.

To test new drugs on humans, pharmaceutical companies must go through a complex four-phase process. According to CenterWatch, the four phases are:

Phase one: Focused on safety. The researchers carefully monitor everyone in the study to find out exactly how the body processes the drug at different dosages. These studies often pay the participants.

Phase two: Concentrates on the effectiveness of the drug. This phase can last a couple of years and typically has several hundred participants. Phase two trials are usually structured as what is known as "blinded"—part of the group gets the drug, part of the group gets a placebo, and no one, researchers or patients, knows who is getting what until the end. About 70 percent of the drugs tested in phase one make it to phase two.

Phase three: This is the intense testing period and involves perhaps several thousand participants. About one-third of newly-proposed drugs make it from phase two to phase three. The drug is thoroughly put through its paces for effectiveness and side effects. This is a very expensive phase for the study sponsor, and interestingly, 90 percent of the drugs that get to this phase do not move on to phase four.

Phase four: Compares the new drug to other therapies for the same condition. Having passed through the other three phases over the course of several years, the drug can also now be monitored for long-term effects.

Participation in a clinical trial is not for everyone. However, everyone with endometriosis could benefit from monitoring what researchers find potentially helpful, in terms of new drugs and new treatment options. Your research could end up being as deep and as vast as that of your doctor, who, besides seeing patients, must also keep up with every disease and condition he and his patients must cope with. So, a good doctor will appreciate your knowledge, especially if you are able to tell her the details of what you've learned. Be sure to note down who did the study, what it found, and where it was printed. If possible, bring her a copy of the study so that she can look at the details.

Your doctor should always respond to your research with respect and interest. If she doesn't, or if you feel she isn't keeping as up-to-date as you would like her, too, be sure to discuss this with her or, if you must, find a new doctor who appreciates the effort you are making in dealing with your illness.

Endometriosis Statistics

You probably have your own personal statistics regarding the time and issues you've dedicated to endometriosis, but research has also come up with a few numbers that you might find interesting regarding the symptoms and medical correlations between endometriosis and other illnesses:

- Seventy-nine percent of women with endometriosis report bowel symptoms.

- Thirty to 40 percent of women with endo experience infertility. (This statistic is not far from women without endometriosis. Around 25% of non endo patients have fertility problems.)

- The depth of infiltration of endometriosis is considered a key factor in the level of pelvic pain.

- Between five and six million women in the United States are estimated to have endometriosis.

- Endo affects all races, socioeconomic groups, and all ages from ten to seventy.

- Before 1921, little information on endometriosis was in any medical literature around the world.

- A study in the early 1980s found no link between endometriosis and tampon use.

- There is an increased risk of endometriosis in first-degree family members (that is, close relatives, such as mothers, sisters, and daughters) of women with endometriosis.

(Sources of statistics: *The Endometriosis Sourcebook*, Ballweg, 1995.)

Things Are Looking Up

There is no question that women with endometriosis have a lot of complex issues to confront. However, as this book shows, things are changing. The tools currently available to combat this disease are better now than they were even just a few years ago. More research is underway that will make future treatment of endometriosis much easier and more definitive. In the meantime, read on—your first, most critical tool for fighting endometriosis is knowledge.

CHAPTER TWO ∽

The Primary Symptoms of Endometriosis

Depending on its severity and symptoms, endometriosis can have a significant toll on the physical, mental, and emotional quality of life. Women with endometriosis need to take an active role in their medical treatment and work closely with doctors to manage the many facets of this complex condition. With an average delay in diagnosis of nine or more years, a patient may seek the counsel of five or more physicians before someone correctly diagnoses and treats her. And, as I mentioned before, even in light of medical advances, laparoscopy is the only way to definitively diagnose endo. Finally, sadly, to date there is no absolute cure for this condition. There are effective methods to provide symptomatic relief, but, of course these remedies can only be used once a physician makes an accurate diagnosis.

As I described in Chapter One, endometriosis is essentially the abnormal migration of uterine lining tissue to other areas of the body.

The resulting symptoms can be wide ranging. This chapter provides information about these symptoms, while subsequent chapters cover treatment options.

The cornucopia of symptoms related to endometriosis often seem totally unrelated, which is one reason doctors misdiagnose so many cases of this disease. On top of that, endometriosis symptoms vary so widely among individual women and range so widely throughout the body that the disease can easily masquerade as several other conditions, such as adenomyosis, appendicitis, ovarian cysts, a bowel obstruction, colon cancer, fibroid tumors, irritable bowel syndrome, ovarian cancer, and pelvic inflammatory disease (PID). Here are some of the primary symptoms that women with endo-metriosis experience:

- Pelvic pain, sometimes acute, sometimes chronic
- Lesions and adhesions
- Lumps on the body
- Irregular, heavy, or painful menstrual cycles
- Bowel-related symptoms, such as blockages and painful bowel movements
- Intestinal and stomach problems
- Painful intercourse
- Back pain
- Infertility
- Miscarriage(s) and/or ectopic (tubal) pregnancy
- Exhaustion
- Emotional symptoms like mood swings, depression, and anxiety

If you experience two or more of these symptoms, either continuously or specifically associated with your period, you should suspect endometriosis. Although you might be afraid of hearing that you have a disease, the truth is that identifying the problem is the first step on the road to managing your symptoms.

So don't hesitate to seek a qualified physician if you suspect you have endometriosis. For most women with endo, simply being diagnosed brings immense relief, emotionally as well as physically. After suffering—often for years—from an unidentified condition with troubling symptoms, you will most likely feel reassured to learn that there are treatment options to alleviate your painful and often life-disrupting symptoms.

Persistent Pain Is Real

Women who suffer from persistent pelvic pain may find that their doctors, as well as their families and friends, don't take their pain seriously. A recent survey of women who suffer from chronic pelvic pain found that 40 percent of the women have been told they exaggerate their pain. But pain is a primary symptom of endometriosis. More importnatly, no matter what it's cause, pain is rarely a figment of the imagination. (And, if it is, that needs to be treated, too.)

Unrelieved pain interferes with how easily you move, how well you sleep, and whether you can get along through the day. If you're in pain, it is difficult to concentrate and think clearly. You stop enjoying things because all you notice is the pain, rather than other elements of your life experience. Then, because of the pain, you can become isolated and unable to spend a lot of time with your friends and family. All of this can lead to feelings of anger, fear, resentment, depression, and anxiety. Physical effects of long-term pain include impaired mobility; gastrointestinal (GI) and lung dysfunctions; increased metabolic rate; a weakened immune system; delayed wound healing; loss of appetite; nausea; and fatigue.

As women with symptoms of endo know, pain can hamper every aspect of life. Your doctor should never be dismissive of your pain; if this happens, your best strategy may be to change doctors. (See Chapter Five for more information about pain management and Chapter Ten for advice on finding and working with doctors.)

To help you understand the role of pain associated with endometriosis, let's look at the common sources and causes of pain.

Sources of Pelvic Pain

When endometrial tissue takes up residence outside of the uterus, pelvic pain is by far the most widely reported symptom and the reason most women initially seek medical attention. Paradoxically, the degree of pain experienced by individual women does not always correlate to their stage of the disease, which is currently graded based on the number of lesions and adhesions observed during surgery.

This classification system was originally designed to predict fertility when a surgeon found endometriosis. However, it is currently being revised to more effectively consider the levels of pain, infertility, and symptoms. For now, the categories are:

Stage I—minimal endo, the lesions are shallow and thin.

Stage II—the disease is deeper within surrounding tissue.

Stage III—Moderate endo with denser lesions mixed with stage I or stage II symptoms.

Stage IV—Severe endo with mostly dense and deep lesions.

In keeping with the puzzling nature of endometriosis, a woman with stage IV disease may experience no symptoms (such as pain), while a stage I patient might be in debilitating pain. Basically, the staging system is a method of communicating between professionals as to the severity of a patient's disease. There are a great many shortcomings to this system, so ask your doctor why he is choosing a particular stage to characterize your illness.

Lesions

As described in Chapter One, during the various stages of the menstrual cycle, the endometrium (the tissue lining the uterus) normally swells and engorges with blood, and then finally sheds in response to hormonal signals. Endometriosis results when bits of endometrial tissue lodge in other areas of the body outside the uterus and continue to respond to the same signals to thicken and then shed just like normal uterine lining tissue. When this tissue is outside of its normal place, there is no passageway for the blood to release and shed, so it must be absorbed by surrounding tissue, which is a comparatively slow process.

Meanwhile, the blood accumulates in body cavities, which can create iternal bleeding, tissue damage, inflammation, and the formation of scar tissue. The cells of this tissue don't always respond to hormones and other bodily functions the way healthy tissues responds, which is one reason it is difficult to predict how a patient will respond to hormone therapy and other treatments.

Women have had endometrial lining wander to just about everywhere in their bodies, with the exception of the spleen. However, it usually finds its way to the ovaries, fallopian tubes, bladder, bowel, appendix, peritoneum (back of abdominal cavity), and the area under and behind the uterus known as the cul-de-sac. As the hormonal cycle recurs month after month, the endometrial tissue implants, also known as lesions, may get bigger and become surrounded by fibrous tissue. In severe cases, connective scar tissue (adhesions) also develops.

When doctors perform diagnostic surgery to find endometriosis, they look for lesions. Lesions take on a variety of forms and colors, ranging from red to brown, black, white, yellow or clear, pink or red. Black lesions are considered typical. Older lesions may seed new lesions and form scar tissue and adhesions (scar tissues that connect organs or other tissues). These inflammatory changes, scarring, and tissue damage can cause significant changes in normal tissues, sometimes leading to infertility.

In other words, the unhealthy tissue can beget more unhealthy tissue and more uncomfortable symptoms. That's why, as is usual when it comes to health, an early, accurate diagnosis is so helpful.

Lesions and adhesions come in a variety of sizes and shapes. There is some evidence that the color, location, and depth of endometrial lesions and adhesions coincide to the degree and types of pain women experience. Research into the relationship between the various classifications of lesions and the pain experienced has been inconclusive, however doctors have anecdotally reported that newer lesions are less likely to have scar tissue covering them and so they may hurt more than older lesions.

Another significant factor in the degree of pain may be the depth of the disease. Some research indicates that lesions which have penetrated more than five millimeters into surrounding tissues seem to correlate to severe pelvic pain. Superficial cysts are less painful. But, there is even an exception to that rule. Some lesions take a lot of abuse and so are more painful. If a lesion is cells that engorge during the monthly cycle or is close to an area of the body that is stimulated during sex, they may hurt a lot, too.

Doctors look very close at how deeply endometriosis has infiltrated specific areas of the body in determining whether surgical intervention is necessary or how extensive their procedure will be. Surface removal of lesions won't end pain if the lesion has penetrated into surrounding tissue. Instead, to provide releif, a doctor must remove or destroy the entire lesion to its full depth.

Adhesions
Adhesions are scar tissues that stretch between two surfaces, connecting areas that would not normally meet. They are one of the many complications that can arise from endometriosis because they can

obstruct, twist, and otherwise impair organs and delicate tissues. Adhesions sometimes block fallopian tubes, causing infertility (as well as pain). And, unfortunately, they can even form after surgery (because they are scar tissue). Even more unfortunately, adhesions don't respond to any treatment except surgery, which means women sometimes need additional surgeries to remove the adhesions.

The pelvic organs, including the ovaries and fallopian tubes are the most common sites for adhesions. Additionally, adhesions can occur on top of an endometrial lesion, which can increase the pressure and pain as well as make the lesion difficult to identify during surgery. Adhesions can also form on or near the diaphragm, the organs in the abdomen, and occasionally even on the lungs, but this is rare.

Adhesions occur in the pelvis because a thin membrane called the peritoneum protects the abdominal cavity and when that membrane suffers damage, such as following surgery, infection, or through a chronic disease process like endometriosis, a sticky protein like substance called fibrin is released on the injured surface. Normally, raw or inflamed tissues form scar tissue to heal, but damaged pelvic tissues covered by fibrin adhere to each other. Because pelvic organs are relatively mobile and can shift, the fibrous scar tissue between surfaces is stretched and elongated by movement, binding organs or adhering them to pelvic sidewalls, causing pain. Lesions can also become trapped within adhesions, making it difficult to detect and remove them.

Surgeons find pelvic adhesions more frequently in moderate to severe endometriosis, but nothing is an absolute with this condition: Pelvic adhesions can also occur with milder endo, too.

Approximately 30 percent of adhesion cases cause problems such as chronic pelvic pain, bowel obstructions, painful intercourse, and even infertility. Adhesive disease accounts for 49 to 74 percent of small bowel obstructions; 15 to 20 percent of infertility cases; and 20 to 50 percent of chronic pelvic pain cases. Adhesions can also complicate future surgical procedures.

Symptoms of adhesions range from acute cramps to chronic pelvic discomfort. Abdominal and pelvic adhesions rarely show up on x-rays or diagnostic tests, and exploratory surgery may be required to identify or rule them out.

I should point out that adhesions are a potential complication of most surgeries, not just surgery related to endometriosis. Of course, doctors have made great progress in preventing the formation of adhesions. They can use several techniques during surgery to prevent them, including infusing certain solutions into the pelvic cavity through the laparoscope, inserting pieces of material such as Gore-Tex into the area, and applying a methylcellulose barrier during surgery. Methyl-cellulose barriers keep surfaces from rubbing together after surgery and have been very effective in reducing post-surgical adhesion formation. These barriers are degradable and the body absorbs them a couple of weeks after surgery, which protects the organs during the time period when most adhesions form. Fortunately, laparoscopic surgery and new adhesion barriers have reduced the chances of adhesion formation quite a lot. To reduce this risk, you must make sure that your surgeon has significant experience in endometriosis surgery specifically. Adhesions are only one of the reasons we cover surgery so extensively in this book.

Endometrial Cysts

Women with endometriosis may be at a higher risk for developing ovarian cysts called endometriomas. These cysts are endometrial cells that grow and bleed in response to estrogen, causing pain. Endometriomas are sometimes called chocolate cysts because they are brown, a result of pooled blood. They range from being quite small to becoming the size of a grapefruit. If a cyst ruptures, it can cause excruciating pain.

Lumps on the Body

Rarely, endometriosis can also appear as lumps in various parts of the body, such as lodged in the skin or in the arms, legs, and even the brain. Women have reported finding lumps in lymph nodes, the lung, heart, eye, armpit, and knee. These lumps may shrink and grow in response to hormonal signals, as is typical of endometrial tissue.

Inflammatory Pain

The lesions of endometriosis, which have both chemical and mechanical roots, contribute to much of the pain from which women with this disease suffer. Internal bleeding, inflammation, and formation of scar tissue are inevitable as endometrial lesions respond to hormonal signals every month.

Endometrial cells release chemicals, such as prostaglandins and histamine, that can cause inflammation. If a endometiral cyst ruptures, these substances flood the surrounding tissues and further irritate the body's pain receptors. Pain receptors seem to become increasingly sensitive to stimulation under the influence of these inflammatory chemicals. Studies show that "message centers" at the site of inflammation, which are called nociceptors, then start to exhibit a lower threshold for pain. Nociceptors normally respond only to strong stimuli, but inflammatory chemicals sensitize them and cause them to transmit pain signals in response to even minimal stimuli.

Normally, prostaglandins contribute to the sloughing of the endometrial lining during menstruation by causing blood vessels and muscles to constrict. However, excessive production of prosta-glandins in the uterine endometrium is linked to pain, cramping, vomiting, and diarrhea during menstruation (see "Painful Periods" on the following page). A prostaglandin known as PGE2 can cause swelling and pain and also thicken the blood, which can lead to congestion and stagnation in the pelvic area. The inflammatory process may also compress or stretch pain receptors in the body.

Scar tissue, a common phenomenon in endometriosis, can deprive pain receptors of oxygen by restricting their access to blood vessels. It may also restrict the usual passage of metabolic wastes, soaking pain receptors in an irritating chemical soup. Pain also results when lesions invade tissues or organs, including the urinary or intestinal tracts.

There is also evidence that endometriosis may exist invisibly at a microscopic level. In *The Endometriosis Sourcebook* (1995), the Edometriosis Association speculates that even before lesions become visible, microscopic endometrial tissue might create a high degree of pelvic inflammation, sending pain signals to the brain along neural pathways that have only recently been charted. Clear, microscopic papules may lodge themselves on the under-side of organs or beneath the skin. Unfortunately, physicians who are less trained to recognize all of the manifestations of edometriosis may miss these diseased areas. So even if no endometriosis is apparent to the surgeon during laparoscopy, samples of tissue should still be taken for biopsy. Pathology results often show evidence of disease in otherwise normal-appearing areas.

Painful Periods

Menstrual periods are often particularly painful for women who have endometriosis. One hundred percent of respondents to an Endometriosis Association questionnaire said they experienced pain one to two days before their periods. Pain is typically felt before and during menstruation. Pain also may develop after several years of pain-free periods.

Often, endometriosis remains undiagnosed for a long time. A symptom such as pain at menstruation may not be seen as unusual, because our culture tends to discount menstrual pain or even see it as normal. However, painful periods, especially when pain is long-term, are not normal.

Recent evidence links severe cramps to excessive production of prostaglandin, the chemical that causes uterine contractions.

Prostaglandin levels normally increase before menstruation, but when the balance of these chemicals is out of sync, the uterine muscles may contract hard enough to restrict normal blood supply to the uterus. Severe pain results when a muscle is deprived of the oxygen normally received through the blood vessels. As a result, cramps may be debilitating and be accompanied by general pelvic or lower-back pain.

Endometriosis sometimes causes premenstrual spotting and progressively heavy menstrual flow. Abnormal bleeding affects about one-third of women with endo. Known as menorrhagia, heavy flow means a loss of about three ounces of blood during a menstrual cycle, double the amount lost during normal cycles. Irregular periods, progressively shorter menstrual cycles, spotting before periods, mid-cycle bleeding, and a dark discharge after a period are other typical menstrual symptoms of endo.

Painful menstruation, also called dysmenorrhea, is common and includes a range of symptoms from pain to diarrhea, nausea, dizziness, and headaches. Pain at ovulation is also possible as lesions respond to hormonal stimulation by bleeding, irritating nerve endings in the pelvis.

Gastrointestinal Endometriosis

Women with endometriosis suffer from intestinal symptoms nearly as much as they do from dysmenorrhea. Endometriosis can implant within the intestines and cause painful bowel movements, lower back pain (especially with periods and with bowel movements), constipation, bloody stools, pressure and a sense of urgency to move the bowels, and even partial or complete obstruction of the bowels. (Fortunately, the worst-case scenario—complete blockage—is rare. However, if bowel movements become impossible, quick medical attention is necessary to relieve blockages.) Digestive symptoms include a swollen abdomen or intestinal gas. In more advanced cases, inflammation may lead to pinched nerve pain. Lesions that invade the small intestine may cause abdominal swelling, pain, and vomiting.

The length of the intestines—five feet for the large intestine and twenty for the small intestine—makes locating and surgically removing intestinal lesions difficult. To complicate matters, even if ovaries are removed to control endometriosis in severe cases, intestinal endo lesions sometimes persist.

Gastrointestinal endometriosis has a long continuum of disease severity from very superficial to very invasive, and some patients can have both superficial disease in one area of the bowel and bulky invasive disease in another. When endometriosis deeply invades the bowel wall, it causes a lot of scarring and can form a tumor that partially obstructs the bowel wall. When the disease is very superficial, it usually causes no symptoms at all. Most patients with GI endometriosis do not have rectal bleeding, although rectal bleeding and painful symptoms occur during the menstrual flow do raise suspicions of GI involvement.

The location of GI endometriosis follows well-defined patterns. The lower rectosigmoid colon is most commonly involved, followed by the last part of the ileum (the small intestine), the cecum (the first part of the large bowel), and the appendix (which hangs off of the cecum). Thirty percent of patients have more than one GI area involved. Superficial disease in any of these areas usually causes no symptoms, but bulky, deeply invasive disease can cause real problems.

A rectal nodule can cause painful bowel movements all month long, rectal pain during intercourse or while sitting, and rectal pain with passing gas. It can also cause constipation, although diarrhea can be present during the menstrual flow. When the sigmoid colon is invaded by bulky disease, patients can have constipation alternating with diarrhea and intestinal bloating and cramping. Bulky endometriosis invading the ileum can result in right lower quadrant pain, bloating, and intestinal cramping. Disease of the cecum and appendix usually causes no specific symptoms at all. Intestinal problems may also stem from adhesions, which may result either from the disease itself or from healing from surgery and are quite common. Abdominal adhesions can cause pain when movement, such as intercourse and pelvic or rectal exams, stretches them. The pain may appear after exercise, during pelvic exams, or be completely unsolicited. Many people describe the pain caused by adhesions as "pulling" or "stabbing," whereas endometriosis pains are often described as "burning" or "pinching."

Adhesions on the bowel can cause a set of symptoms all their own, including pain, nausea, irritable bowel syndrome, and occasionally intestinal blockage. Bowel obstructions and bladder problems can be consequences of pelvic adhesions, and corrective surgery is sometimes indicated. In cases of intestinal involvement, nausea, bloating, abdominal distention, and vomiting can occur. If you experience a sudden inability to pass fecal matter or gas and are very ill with nausea or vomiting, see your physician immediately to rule out a bowel obstruction.

The Prostaglandin Connection

Lesions or adhesions in the bowels do not directly cause all of the gastrointestinal symptoms of endometriosis. When symptoms—including diarrhea, nausea, vomiting, and general intestinal discomfort—are at their worst during the menstrual period, chalk it up to a prostaglandin imbalance. These biochemicals control the smooth tissues of the involuntary muscles. They trigger uterine contractions, control blood vessel diameter, and regulate intestinal function. Excessive uterine prostaglandin production causes severe period cramping, and it can also affect other smooth muscles in the body when the extra prostaglandin secreted by endometrial tissues enters the bloodstream. Intestinal muscles contract too quickly, leading to pain and diarrhea. Blood vessels may constrict and dilate, causing many women with endometriosis to feel cold or to experience hot flashes.

Candidiasis

Another set of intestinal symptoms that women with endometriosis frequently endure are related to candidiasis, an infection caused by a common yeast-like fungus, Candida albicans. This fungus is normally present in the mouth, throat, vagina, and intestines in balance with other bacteria and yeasts in the body. It becomes problematic if a pH imbalance causes the fungus to multiply, creating long branches of yeast cells known as candidiasis.

The long list of possible symptoms of candidiasis includes constipation, diarrhea, colitis, abdominal pain, headaches, bad breath, rectal itching, mood swings, memory loss, facial numbness, night sweats, clogged sinuses, white spots on the tongue and mouth (thrush), pre-menstrual syndrome (PMS), extreme fatigue, vaginitis, urinary tract infections, arthritis, depression, heartburn, sore throat, hyperthyroidism, and adrenal problems. In severe cases, Candida can travel through the bloodstream and invade other organ systems, causing a type of blood poisoning called Candida septicemia.

Candidiasis is frequently evident in people with compromised immune systems and is often accompanied by food and environmental allergies. Another contributing factor is prolonged or frequent antibiotic use, which weakens the immune system and causes an imbalance between the Candida bacteria and the "friendly" bacteria that normally control Candida, thus allowing Candida to multiply. Many women with gastrointestinal symptoms have found relief through treatment of candidiasis, including nutritional strategies and other approaches to strengthening their immune systems. Recent research into endometriosis is finding evidence of the importance of the immune system in the development and management of endometriosis. (See Chapter Seven to learn more about the role of the body's immune system in related endometrial conditions and for natural strategies for enhancing immune system function.)

Urinary Tract Symptoms
Occasionally, the bladder also becomes an endometriosis host. Symptoms are similar to those of urinary tract infections: abdominal

pain, painful urination, frequent need to urinate, and urinary retention. There may also be blood in the urine during menstruation.

Adhesions can also exert pressure on the bladder or involve the ureters, the ducts that carry urine from the kidneys to the bladder. If endometriosis obstructs the ureters, the risk of kidney failure necessitates aggressive treatment, including surgery. High blood pressure may develop when ureters are blocked, so women with endometriosis who experience hypertension should seek diagnosis for endo involvement in the urinary tract.

Symptoms of interstitial cystitis (IC) are similar to those listed above and are frequently noted in women with endo. If you are diagnosed with IC, therefore, ask your doctor to evaluate you carefully for the possible presence of endometriosis.

Painful Sex

Surveys of women with endometriosis find that 59 percent experience painful sex, most often related to the size and location of endometrial lesions or adhesions. When any area of the reproductive tract that is stretched, pushed, or pulled by the activity of intercourse has been invaded by lesions or adhesions, penetrating sex may be acutely painful. Cul-de-sac (the membranous wall between the rectum and the vagina) endo is a known culprit for causing painful intercourse, particularly upon deep penetration.

For some women, orgasms are also painful. Women report sometimes feeling pain after sex that may last more than a day. Sex may be more painful at specific times during the hormonal cycle or in specific positions.

Another problem for women with endometriosis may be vaginal dryness, a by-product of some hormone therapies. If the ovaries have been removed, vaginal dryness and atrophy due to low estrogen may further contribute to painful sex. Loss of sex drive (libido) is also a common consequence of surgical removal of ovaries.

Many women report that treating endometriosis eliminates or reduces the pain they experience during sex. However, because endo is chronic, when lesions return, pain often does, too.

Back Pain

About one-third of all women with endometriosis experience back pain. This is yet another symptom than many women don't connect to their endo until they have a diagnosis.

Low back pain that radiates or travels to the buttock and upper thigh is the most cited problem. Studies have shown that endo can invade the sciatic nerve, which can, at the same time, be affected by the general inflammation and muscle spasms typical of endo. Symptoms include pain that begins just before menstruation and lasts several days after the end of the flow, low back discomfort radiating to the left leg, left foot weakness, cramping in the left leg when walking for long distances, and tenderness of the sciatic notch.

If women focus solely on their back pain and don't treat their endometriosis, the symptoms become less cyclical over time, due to scarring and the creation of new lesions. This results in a progressively shorter pain-free interval until constant pain prevails. Early recognition prevents permanent damage to the sciatic nerve. Additionnally, adenomyosis (a condition related to endometriosis) causes back pain symptoms.

Infertility

Because endometriosis primarily strikes the reproductive organs, infertility is a common outcome. Approximately one-third of infertility patients are diagnosed with endometriosis, and approximately one-third of women with endo are considered infertile. Some asymptomatic women don't discover that they have the disease until they try to conceive and have difficulty. These perceived difficulties may not be as significant as once thought, though, and most women with endo have similar pregnancy rates as their peers without endometriosis.

Endometriosis can contribute to infertility in several ways. Scar tissue may block the fallopian tubes or interfere with ovulation. In severe cases, when adhesions are formed, infertility results because the motility of the tubes is reduced. In less severe cases, the increased production of prostaglandin by the endometriosis probably interferes with normal tubal and ovarian function.

Another result of endometriosis is the formation of ovarian cysts called endometrioma that may also interfere with ovulation. And since the goal of many hormone treatments for endo is to curtail ovulation, treatment itself often contributes to infertility, at least temporarily.

Chapter Nine will look in depth at infertility causes and concerns, incl-uding miscarriages and ectopic pregnancy risks.

Energy Deficits

The reasons that women with endometriosis often have low energy levels and exhaustion are multi-layered and intertwined. It's likely that these debilitating symptoms are related to the autoimmune processes of the disease and exacerbated by the body's reactions to constant inflammation and to the increased physical, mental, and emotional stress from dealing with chronic pain.

Women with endometriosis commonly report that pain interferes with sleep. Seventy-eight percent reported difficulty falling asleep because of pain or being awakened from sleep by pain. This finding is significant because fatigue tends to increase the severity of pain.

Acute insomnia may flare before or after a surgery, due to anxieties and/or physical pain. Medications may also increase or cause insomnia. One of the known side effects of some drugs used to treat endometriosis, such as GnRHs (see Chapter Three), is insomnia.

Depression—which is a common addendum to any chronic disease, particularly a disease that causes pain—can certainly be associated with complaints of lack of energy. Any assessment regarding this debilitating process must account for the psycho-physiologic effects of the endometriosis which are well known.

Emotional Effects

Living with endometriosis undoubtedly puts women under high levels of stress. Issues that travel hand-in-hand with endo—such as chronic pain, worries over health, infertility, relationship troubles, sexual concerns, job security, financial worries, and so on—challenge self-esteem and sabotage feelings of well-being. Unfortunately, stress itself can worsen pain and increase muscle tension, which decreases blood circulation and oxygenation to the pelvic area.

Fluctuating hormones normally trigger mood swings in women of reproductive age; for women with endometriosis, these expected swings can be both higher and lower than usual. Also, many of the hormonal drugs used to combat endometriosis can contribute to unreliable and uneven moods, sometimes including depression.

Maintaining emotional health while living with endometriosis is an immense challenge. Many women report intense guilt feelings about not being able to participate fully as partners and mothers in the lives of their families. A more positive outlook may seem easier some days than others. Make time during your better days for pleasures, simple or grand. On the not-so-good days, allowing yourself to occasionally just stay in bed to "enjoy" some self-indulgence or self-pity can be therapeutic. Suppressing deeply felt emotions increases stress; venting can be just the thing!

If the emotional weight becomes more than you can bear, seek support from health professionals, friends, or other women with endometriosis. Sometimes the best way to figure out how to take care of yourself in the midst of this disease is by talking to others with endometriosis.

Many natural approaches to endo care have improved women's responses to both the physical disease and the emotional side effects of living with endo. Chapter Seven reviews some natural treatments to help you get through some of the emotional side effects of endometriosis, and Chapter Eleven describes some ways to get the support you need from friends, family, and more formal outlets such as support groups and online chat rooms.

There IS Hope!

The list of symptoms for a chronic and complex condition like endometriosis can be daunting. But there is a bright side: Once you have a diagnosis, you can see how some of the seemingly unrelated issues you've been dealing with fit into a complex puzzle. From there, you can make some changes to create a more pain-free life. Knowledge is power—keep learning!

CHAPTER THREE ❧

Drugs and Other Therapies

Endometriosis logically should be treatable using some sort of systemic therapy, since it is predominantly a pelvic disorder that can occasionally spread or occur in other areas of the body. Also, although it is not cancer, many doctors have likened endometriosis to a cancerous growth because of how it spreads and invades other parts of the body. It would be logical then to treat the disease with the equivalent of "chemotherapy" in the form of medicine or other types of non-surgical and holistic approaches. I'll explain some of these approaches and whether these types of treatments have been successful.

What Is The Goal of Treatment?

Before we get into the details of treatment, I think it is important to discuss its goals. Doctors treat endometriosis symptomatically, which means that it is their goal to reduce the patient's symptoms, sometimes separate from each other. For example, a doctor may focus on both the pain and the potential for infertility. One reason for this is that, to date, I am unaware of any evidence that any mode of therapy—whether it be surgery, medicine, or holistic methods—has resulted in an endometriosis cure. Therefore, the goal is to get rid of the symptoms for as long as possible with as few side effects.

Pain Relievers

Pain is the number one problem for the majority of endometriosis sufferers. Painful periods, pain at mid-cycle, and pain during and after sexual relations are the most common complaints from women who suffer with endometriosis. Other common problems include irritable bowel symptoms (nausea, diarrhea, gas, constipation, cramping, etc.), irritable bladder symptoms (urinary frequency, urgency, burning, stinging, etc.), fibromyalgia, depression, chronic fatigue syndrome, and infertility. Since some type of pain is the most common symptom and all of the other problems mentioned above are in a way related to pain, let's first talk about solutions to this complaint.

Doctors can treat pain in several ways. First, they can use drugs, most commonly analgesics. These medications work in a variety of ways but their goals are the same: They reduce the perceived painful response. The group most people are familiar with is NSAIDs (non-steroidal anti-inflammatory drugs). NSAIDs include Motrin and Aspirin. NSAIDs work by reducing the circulating level of substances called prostaglandins. Prostaglandins are chemicals in the bloodstream that are associated with pain. As explained in Chapter Two, prostaglandins contribute to the sloughing of the endometrial lining during menstruation by causing blood vessels and muscles to constrict. But en-dometriosis can cause the body to make too much prostaglandin, and greater levels of prostaglandins mean greater pain.

NSAIDs are quite safe and are generally effective, at least at first, in reducing or eliminating pain from endometriosis. The only side effect of these medicines is that they can at times cause stomach pain. Therefore, they are not recommended for people who have reflux (GERD, or gastro-esophageal reflux disease) or stomach ulcers. Stronger pain medicines are available, but all of these drugs are controlled substances (narcotics). Doctors try very hard to limit the use of these drugs in this situation because of a strong potential for abuse and addiction. Muscle relaxants may be prescribed simultaneously with other drugs because their sedative effect often enhances the pain-reducing effects of the NSAID or narcotic analgesics.

A number of other medications may be used for chronic pain. These medications aren't solely used for pain reduction and may be prescribed in what is called an "off-label" manner. This means that the drug or treatment has been approved by the U.S. Food and Drug Administration (FDA) for a particular situation but that the drug has not been FDA-approved for the specific use in this case. The best example of off-label prescriptions is the use of antidepressants to treat chronic pain. Also, studies have shown that anti-epileptic drugs can be successful in reducing pain.

Other Drugs

The FDA must approve drugs for various uses. Generally, this agency is like a lumbering giant: it does a very good job of not allowing any drug that has potential harm to the public to become available in the United States, but the approval process is very slow and arduous and it costs an enormous amount of money to get a drug approved for sale in this country. The stringency of the FDA process to approve any therapy which involves drugs or devices is not without flaws. The researchers involved with testing new therapies are all certainly experts in the field, but they're sometimes are not on the front lines of patient care. Therefore, sometimes questions that could have been answered during the drug trials remain unanswered even up until the time that the drug hits the shelf. Medical professionals are stuck trying to answer these questions for their patients without adequate data. A number of drugs over the years have been approved by the FDA for use in the treatment of endometriosis. Virtually all of these drugs use hormonal manipulation in some way to improve endometriosis symptoms. And virtually all of these drugs have been developed in the last twenty-five years.

If you look at the history of the development of these medicines, you'll find that many of the medicines were designed based on incorrect assumptions and myths about the causes and "cures" of endometriosis. Early on, researchers found that women who became pregnant were "cured" of their endometriosis. These observations brought about the earliest "pseudo-pregnancy" treatments for the disease.

In this general field would be the use of Depo-Provera, birth control pills (BCPs), and continuous progesterone hormone therapy. These treatments have been relatively successful in reducing pain in certain women, particularly if the menstrual periods are suppressed. Also, it was observed that endometriosis regressed or got better after "the change" had occurred and, thus, the "pseudo-menopause" treatments

Type of Medication	Brand Name	Symptom Relief	Side Effects	Cost
Acetaminophen	Tylenol, Panadol	Minimal relief	Very rare	Cheap, over the counter (OTC)
NSAIDs (non-steroidal anti-inflamma-tory drugs)	Motrin, Aleve, Advil, Anaprox, Vioxx, Celebrex	Moderate relief	GI upset, raises blood pressure.	Cheap if generic OTC; expensive if by prescription
Pseudo-pregnancy	Depo-Provera, Nor-lutate, Aygestin	Moderate relief	Spotting, fluid retention, weight gain	Moderate price (prescription)
Birth control pills— continuous/ sequential	Ortho Novum, Lo/Ovral, Loestrin, etc.	Moderate relief	Spotting, fluid retention, weight gain	Moderate price
Pseudo-menopausal	Danazol, Lupron, Zoladex	Can provide excellent relief	Risks of menopause (cardiovascu-lar & osteoporosis), mood swings, hot flashes, hair loss	Expensive; requires injection or placement (Lupron and Zoladex)
Anti-seizure medications	Tegretol, Neurontin	Enhances relief	Multiple, including birth defects	Moderate to expensive
Antidepressants	Elavil, Tofranil, Prozac, Serafem, Zoloft, Paxil	May enhance relief	Poorly understood mechanism of action but few side effects are known	Moderate

were born. The initial pseudo-menopause drug was Danazol. Now our efforts in this field revolve around what are called gonadotropin agonists (GnRH, under the brand names of Lupron, Synarel, etc), gonadotropin antagonists (no approved drug yet), and aromatase inhibitors (Femara). All of these drugs seek through various hormonal methods to lower circulating estrogen. Of course, researchers now know that endometriosis does exist in post-menopausal women, but active growth of endo probably subsides when women reach their late thirties and forties. Androgen treatment (male hormone) has also been used, but success in this area is quite variable. I should remind you, though, that there are still no known medical/drug therapies that eliminate or cure endometriosis.

Of all of these treatments, the GnRH agonist (Lupron) has generated the most discussion. There is even a web site called the Lupron Victims Network, supposedly meant to aid those patients who have had problems with this drug. I'd like to say this about drug therapy in general: of those doctors who treat endometriosis seriously on a daily basis, each of us has had success using one or more of the treatments mentioned here and each of us have had failures. Any drug or treatment has a potential for side effects and also the potential of failing to treat the symptoms intended to be helped. The most important thing you can do is to become as informed as possible and ask your practitioner detailed questions about whatever the proposed treatment may be. Yes, Lupron may cause hot flashes, mood swings, memory loss, bone loss, and decreased sex drive. But if it eliminates incapacitating pain and if it can be combined with other medicines that can eliminate some of those side effects (this treatment is called Lupron + add-back therapy and is recognized by the FDA as a valid treatment for endometriosis), then Lupron could be the right choice for some women.

As a doctor who treats endometriosis, I strongly believe that we need every potential therapy to help the large group of women who suffer from this disease on a daily basis. I cannot simply rule out a drug regimen if that treatment might be appropriate and effective for even one of my patients. Remember that our goal is to treat the symptoms of the disease since we don't have a cure.

Danazol or Danocrine is a synthetic testosterone (male hormone). It works in some ways like Lupron but has some unique side effects that are attributed to the male derivation of the drug. In addition to menopause-like symptoms, some people taking Danazol will develop acne, voice deepening, and hair loss if on the medication for prolonged periods. These effects are dose related and have for the most part been eliminated by going to lower dosages of the medication. The original recommended dose of 800 mg per day has been reduced to less than half that dosage, and patients are doing better with the medication with decreased side effects. Add-back therapy with Danazol has not been approved by the FDA, but there is some activity in this area that could improve some of the menopausal side effects (hot flashes, mood swing, etc.).

The other hormone treatments have side effects that are common among women who take oral contraceptives (BCPs) and similar medicines. Some women have weight gain, swelling, nausea, and mood disturbances from these medications. These symptoms occur in less than 10 percent of women taking this type of treatment, and, at times, very acceptable levels of pain relief are achieved.

So, all of these treatments are, at some level, double-edged swords. They may have side effects, but the potential for pain reduction may be sufficient enough that it's worth taking a chance that the side effects will be bearable. Also, virtually all the treatments described here have no lasting effects beyond the time that the medications are taken. In other words, if you have fluid retention on BCPs, the fluid will disappear when you stop taking them.

A couple of other comments about BCPs are in order. First, they provide excellent birth control for those people not wishing to conceive. At the same time, of course, they are not particularly useful for treating endometriosis if a woman is seeking pregnancy. Second, the effect of BCPs is predominately that of "quieting" the pelvis, decreasing menstrual flow, or eliminating menstrual flow. Ovulation (egg production) should cease for optimal effect of these drugs. This means that certain types of BCPs are better than others in this case. Monophasic pills (Loestrin, OrthoCyclen, Lo/Ovral, Alesse) are best in this regard, although many of the newest brands of BCPs are triphasic (Ortho TriCyclen, Trophasil, Trinorinyl).

Many times, doctors treating endometriosis prescribe BCPs to be taken in a continuous fashion rather than a sequential manner. This means that a woman would take active pills every day of the month (with no cycle of the inactive pills that are typically included in a month's dosage of BCPs) in an effort to stop bleeding altogether. I am frequently asked if this is harmful in any way. The answer is simply "no." Absence of bleeding, if induced in this way, causes no harm and certainly can decrease or eliminate endo pain. As usual, this benefit can be associated with other side effects. Most common with continuous BCP treatment is "break-through bleeding," or spotting in between periods. This effect is caused by the suppression of hormonal effects on the uterine lining, which can make the lining too thin, making it unstable and likely to fall off. This is seen as spotting. To treat this problem, the patient is simply given a little extra estrogen to take with her BCPs each day for about a month, which usually eliminates spotting by thickening the uterine lining and decreasing its instability. I always liken this situation to paint on the ceiling: if the paint gets too thin and dry, it will curl and flake off. To stop this, you apply multiple coats of paint to the ceiling, thus thickening and stabilizing it. Estrogen has the same effect on the uterine lining.

Other Treatments
So-called holistic therapies have also been used in the treatment of pain from endometriosis. These therapies include dietary regimens as well as herbal medicines, which have all achieved some success in pain reduction. (See Chapter Seven for a more complete discussion on alternative therapies, including those for pain management.)

Diets that are meat-free, high protein, high carbohydrate, low carbohydrate, macrobiotic, low fat, or "natural," and every other alteration in diet, have been recommended for pain relief. Variable results have been obtained. It does seem that women who are closer to their ideal weight for their body type are less likely to be affected by pain syndromes. Herbal remedies such as black cohosh, ginseng, and licorice have all been used, and some who use these agents have reported relief of symptoms. Other as-yet-unreported botanicals may at some point become recognized treatments for pain disorders like endometriosis. The great thing about the vast majority of these substances is that they have so little potential for harm. Few, if any, people will be hurt trying these botanicals. If there is a down side to the use of these therapies, it is that they could distract women from known effective therapies.

One potential pain relief treatment is the use of your own biochemical factory to treat yourself. Endorphins (biochemical "good guys" produced by the brain) are manufactured in response to exercise and can serve as a pain reducer/reliever in women with pelvic pain due to endometriosis. Although doctors don't completely understand how endorphins are produced, we do know that endorphins are potent pain relievers that use the same pathway as the narcotic morphine. We also know that endorphins can be addictive, but they can be seen as a positive addiction that encourages us to exercise. For pain relief from endorphins to be effective, the exercise must be thirty minutes or more of continuous exercise, as vigorous as possible, at least three days per week. Women with endometriosis who exercise according to these guidelines definitely have less pain with menses, and less menstrual bleeding and suffer from fewer PMS symptoms than do women who are less active.

As team doctor to the University of Georgia Women's Athletic Teams, I compared 125 student athletes with a similar group of non-athlete college students of similar backgrounds. In the athletic group (daily workouts, vigorous activity), the absence of pain with periods and in general was remarkable compared to the non-athletes. Five percent of athletes reported pain as compared to 35 percent of non-athletes. The only possible explanation for this significant difference was the activity level in the athletic group.

The best part of exercise therapy is that it is free. The only cost is time. Certainly, limiting your intake of stimulants like caffeine and taking a multivitamin plus minerals (especially zinc, magnesium, and calcium) are helpful, but the addition of regular exercise when possible can be very helpful in the treatment of pain and chronic depressive disorders. A large number of scientific studies have demonstrated positive effects of diet, vitamins, and exercise, and therefore, standard treatment should include exercise and a change in diet, if possible, along with other types of therapy.

The use of massage therapy has been successful in treating pain and may have many therapeutic benefits. Whether you choose deep tissue or shiatsu techniques, massage therapy certainly can be conducted with success. In my experience, acupressure and acupuncture have also proved helpful. The general rule of thumb with this type of treatment is that the practitioner is the most important ingredient. That is, the person who administers the remedy is more critical than the actual type of treatment. Forexample, I have had great success with certain acupuncturists who treat my patients and less success with others. It is best to consult with others and take those recommendations with you to your initial interview with this type of practitioner. Try to achieve a level of comfort with them, as you would with any other caregiver. As with any mode of holistic or, for that matter, traditional medical treatments, there is a certain amount of "placebo effect." This means that a certain number of people will get better for reasons that are unrelated to the specific therapy being used. In addition, the more that interpersonal relations are involved, the greater the placebo effect. I don't mean that these treatments are fraudulent in any way. The placebo effect is just an observed phenomenon that occurs with any type of holistic, medical, or surgical therapy.

Unrelated Symptoms

I should mention that a woman with endometriosis can have symptoms that are not caused by the endo but seem related. The most common symptom is bleeding. This may include regular periods that are excessively heavy or light, bleeding in between regular periods, absence of periods, and constant bleeding. Any or all of these things are considered to be abnormal uterine bleeding (AUB). AUB should never be ignored or simply blamed on endometriosis. A pelvic ultrasound, endometrial biopsy (a scraping sample of the uterine lining, formerly called a D&C), and possibly a hysteroscopy (a procedure described in detail in Chapter Four) should be done to assure that there are no changes in the lining of the uterus that are pre-cancerous or cancerous. After there is adequate explanation that there is no malignancy, medical treatment should be used. Fortunately, many of the hormonal treatments used to decrease the pain of endometriosis are effective in controlling AUB, so both problems can often be addressed with a single medical therapy. Also, sometimes a woman with endometriosis may undergo a conservative surgical procedure that leaves the uterus, fallopian tubes, and ovaries present but may still require medical treatment for control of AUB or may need birth control, so oral contraceptives may be used.

Hormone Replacement

One other area of concern is the question of hormone replacement in a woman who has had surgical removal of both ovaries and who has endometriosis. As discussed in Chapter Four, it is imperative that all visible endometriosis be removed at the time of surgery or the symptoms related to the endometriosis will likely remain.

If the endometriosis is removed, however, there is no reason not to use traditional hormone replacement for these women. Estrogen therapy is indicated and in most cases recommended in women who are young and can benefit from the positive effects of estrogen on the cardiovascular system (the heart) and on the bones (prevention of osteoporosis). For my patients, I most frequently prescribe a combination of estrogen and a very small amount of testosterone that can be taken as a pill or applied to the skin as a cream. Hormone replacement is a controversial issue these days, but in the case of young women who have had their ovaries removed, the benefits of this therapy are far greater than any theoretical risks. The benefits of estrogen remain unquestioned while the suggested risks of breast cancer, for example, are theoretical at best.

The use of progesterone as a component of hormone therapy has recently raised some questions suggesting a moderating effect on the positive aspects of estrogen therapy alone. Even in the situation where progesterone seems appropriate, however, hormonal therapy appears appropriate. The improvement of quality of life as shown in many studies warrants this treatment.

No Cure, Lots of Treatment Options

So, there are many methods and reasons for the use of different medical treatments for endometriosis. Again, unfortunately, there are no known medical cures for endometriosis. There is, however, the possibility of relief of pain, the major symptom involved with the disease. Pain is an extremely difficult problem for anyone, patient or doctor, to handle.

As noted above, a careful assessment of your unique symptoms, along with a physical exam, should point the way for your medical practitioner to improve your quality of life. Take time to talk with your caregivers, ask all the questions you need to understand your treatment plan, and be responsible for getting the treatment that you desire. I have found that when communication is absent, excellence in care is denied. Philosophically speaking, the sooner that everyone in the United States becomes an informed consumer of his/her health care, then the sooner our health care system will itself become healthy again. We still have the best system in the world, but it could use a little doctoring too, and the best surgeons for that task are the patients themselves.

A PERSONAL STORY

Kim

Kim has the classic tale of endometriosis: "I'd always had problems with my periods. They weren't so bad in high school, but I attributed that to the fact that I was very athletic, and I know that exercise helps with period pain and regularity." But Kim got married shortly after high school and her symptoms went downhill from there. Her periods began to get worse, and she had regular infections.

Not classic to the tale, however, is that Kim suspected she had endometriosis. Her doctor kept saying, "No, you don't have the symptoms."

In 1995, she moved from the south to Iowa and, continuing to have problems, went to a new doctor. This doctor immediately said, "You have endometriosis." He scheduled her for surgery, which took several hours. The diagnosis was confirmed, and he cleared out as much of the endometrial lesions as he could.

Kim's doctor told her that, with the recent surgery, now would be the opportune time to get pregnant. He said that she would most likely need more surgery in the future, but that her fallopian tubes were not blocked. She and her husband tried for 18 months, but she could not get pregnant. They gave up trying. Eventually, they divorced and Kim moved back to Georgia.

By then, her periods were so bad that the pain would cause her to vomit. Some months she was rushed to the hospital twice in one day to deal with the pain.

Kim had surgery again. It took a very long time. Her appendix was on the verge of rupturing and was removed. She was excited, thinking that she was going to get much better; instead she got worse, which was, she admits, very discouraging.

She then began taking pain medications. "I tried everything—Percocet, Demerol, everything. I would only build up an immunity until it didn't work anymore. It used to be gradual pain, but now I was just doubling over while just walking down the hall. No position was comfortable. I couldn't do anything—I was bedridden and drugged up for several days each month."

A doctor then gave Kim a prescription for morphine—and she was in so much pain that she took it. Then she started taking it when she didn't need it, which finally led her to realize that morphine wasn't a good choice for her in any situation.

Kim had tried birth control pills to no avail. "In 1998, Dr. Lyons decided we should try Lupron." Lupron is a synthetic gonadotropin-releasing hormone. This type of hormone occurs naturally in the body. Lupron is prescribed in endometriosis patients to suppress the shedding of the uterine lining, to relieve pain, and to reduce the endometrial lesions elsewhere in the body. It basically causes your body to act in ways associated with peri-menopause.

Kim's doctor told her that a lot of women have a hard time with the side effects of Lupron and warned her that she may not be able to take the mental effects of Lupron. Kim thought, "I've been through so much else, what could hurt?"

In fact, for the first couple of months, Kim had severe mood swings. Her parents were ready to call the doctor themselves and beg him to take her off the drug. "I almost couldn't stand myself. Not only the mood swings, but I'd have severe hot flashes. I would be in the grocery store and suddenly feel like I was going to spontaneously combust. I'd head to the frozen foods section!"

Kim's doctor added a small dose of estrogen to help level out Lupron's effects. After a couple of months, Kim's body settled into the new hormonal makeup and the side effects dissipated.

"Finally, for once, I could see a light at the end of the tunnel." She felt great for several years. But then she started getting some break-through bleeding. And things started to go downhill again.

Now 34, Kim is not giving up her lifelong hope of having a child. The pain is worse than ever, but she has started to learn how to head it off a little by using Motrin or like medicines so it can be more bearable. And she is headed back to the doctor to see what the next course of action should be.

Kim feels that no matter what, women with endometriosis should not give up trying to gain control of this disease. "When I would get to my lowest points," she says, "I would think 'you could always be worse off.' I have a home, a job, a great family and colleagues."

"At times you will want to pull your hair out by the roots, but be open to what the doctor recommends and wants to try."

CHAPTER FOUR ∾

Surgical Options

In the last chapter, I discussed the pros and cons of medical therapy for endometriosis. Unfortunately, my experience with medical therapy for symptom relief has been mixed. This chapter covers an area in which I am much more comfortable—relief from endometriosis through surgery.

It's not so much that I am more comfortable with this treatment option because I am a surgeon; rather, I have experience and solid data from our medical center that makes this an easier subject for me to app-roach. I have been treating patients with endometriosis for about 25 years. Over the years, I have found a number of things that consistently seem to work with my patients.

Once Again, the Pain Factor

As you know, the main symptom of endometriosis is pain—pain with intercourse, pain with menstrual periods, pain at mid-cycle, and just pain in general. Besides pain, other symptoms of endometriosis include problems with becoming pregnant and problems staying pregnant once you conceive. Irritable bowel symptoms, irritable bowel syndrome (IBS), and irritable bladder can also be related to endometriosis; 8 percent of the endo patients that come into our clinic complain of some type of IBS symptoms, and almost as many have irritable bladder symptoms. Interstitial cystitis, a disease associated with painful bladder symptoms, is considered by many to be a close associate of endometriosis. Fibromyalgia and chronic fatigue syndrome are also commonly seen in patients with endo.

Why Surgery?

So why is a surgical solution considered to be effective in this complex situation? An excellent question, but unfortunately there is no simple answer.

Through the years, endometriosis has been treated as a disease that affects the whole body (systemic), although it seems that in the vast majority of cases endo is a localized disorder. This means that although the symptoms of this disease are most often global in scope, endometrial lesions and adhesions are usually limited to the area of the lower abdominal cavity. Even though we often hear about it because it is quite phenomenal, only rarely will endometriosis move out of the pelvis to other, more distant sites. Despite the fact that some of the symptoms are relatively systemic, the disease still resides mainly in the pelvis.

If, therefore, we can isolate and remove the disease in the pelvic area, then perhaps we can limit all those symptoms elsewhere. This has proven to be true in my experience, particularly with patients who have symptoms of IBS. After the pelvic endometriosis is taken out through surgery, patients' bowel-related symptoms frequently cease to be as significant. There is no logical explanation for this elimination of symptoms, but the data suggests that this is a real phenomenon. Certainly, fertility improves slightly with excision of endo, even though there appears to be no logical explanation as to why or whether endo makes conception less likely.

Historically, doctors began by using surgery to remove the endometriosis; then, when sophisticated hormonal manipulation became available, we switched more to medical therapy. After finding the limitations of medical therapy in the mid and late 1980s, the medical field has moved back to surgical removal as our chief type of treatment for this baneful disease. Surgeons currently have the ability to do endo surgery in a minimally invasive manner, using the laparoscope and tiny incisions. This approach has numerous advantages. Now surgical treatment for endo usually involves outpatient procedures with very short recovery times performed by surgeons who have a lot of experience with the disease and solid expertise in the field of laparoscopic surgery. It is very important to add here that surgery for endometriosis is technically difficult. Successful surgery frequently is as dependent on the surgeon as on the volume or severity of the disease.

What First?
Many women go for a routine exam and, after giving a history of painful periods, are given the diagnosis of endometriosis without having the doctor suggest the necessary exploratory surgery. Since

many people equate this diagnosis with absolute infertility and a requirement for hysterectomy, the psychological impact can be devastating. Many women and, unfortunately, their doctors assume that the diagnosis of endometriosis limits and restricts women to being barren and needing a major surgical procedure. This simply is not so. It is important to know that there are options that offer hope for virtually all women with endometriosis.

First, a reliable diagnosis of endometriosis can be made only by visual inspection and/or biopsy of the lesions. This means that although you and your doctor may suspect endo, the first step should be to see if medical therapy helps. If endo is suspected, then, you should first receive a round of NSAIDs (non-steroidal anti-inflammatory drugs, such as ibuprofen) and hormonal suppression (birth control pills) if you are able to take them.

Some women can't tolerate birth control pills or hormone management in general, but those whose symptoms improve may continue with this treatment indefinitely. Many times, this medical treatment completely resolves the pain. If the pain is reduced or eliminated, then the medical treatment should be continued as long as it is effective and well-tolerated.

What About Fertility?

At the same time, women with endometriosis should be reassured that their fertility is likely intact and will remain so. If a woman desires to attempt pregnancy, hormone treatment is not appropriate and surgical alternatives must be discussed. Be assured that there is no need for the removal of the uterus, fallopian tubes, or ovaries to treat endometriosis. Particularly for women in their teens and twenties, I do not feel that hysterectomy or even oophorectomy (removal of the ovaries) is an appropriate alternative. There are some rare patients who have severe disease and have completed their childbearing or choose not to try pregnancy in whom uterine removal may be considered, but in general this is not the correct option.

If in the early evaluation large ovarian cysts have been found on ultrasound or other factors such as bowel symptoms have been noted, you could be told that any surgery will require a larger abdominal incision (laparotomy). This also is not necessarily true, as virtually all procedures for endometriosis can be done through laparoscopic surgery. Therefore, look for laparoscopic options from the doctor—if they are not presented to you, ask why.

Many times, the reason for the advised laparotomy is because of the potential for cancer in a woman who has a "complex adnexal mass." Doctors then often order a blood test called a CA 125. However, this test should never be done on a woman who is pre-menopausal because the results of the test are not applicable to this age group of women. Again, laparoscopy remains the best way to care for a woman with endo, no matter what the situation. In this case, elevated CA 125 would demonstrate clearly that endo was present, not cancer of the ovary.

Why Is Endometriosis Best Treated by Laparoscopy?

There are several reasons why endo is best treated using the laparoscope:

- The most common findings with endometriosis are minimal or moderate disease. These changes are at times very difficult to see and require the magnification that laparoscopy offers.

- The position of the disease in the pelvis is such that it is almost impossible to clearly see the disease process using a traditional abdominal incision, no matter how large the incision. Most of the areas of endometriosis occur in the posterior area of the pelvic cavity called the cul-de-sac.

- Sometimes in severe situations with disease occurring in distant sites such as the diaphragm, the laparoscope enables the surgeon to see all of these areas and to treat all of the endometriosis through several tiny incisions less than a dime in size.

- The relative risk of scar tissue occurring after laparoscopy is significantly less than with traditional surgery. Since we know that this risk is decreased, and since we also know that scarring or adhesions can cause pain, logically we would prefer the laparoscopic approach over traditional large-incision surgery.

Adhesions are less likely to form after laparoscopic surgery for several reasons. First, the risk of bleeding is significantly less in laparoscopic procedures. Blood is a potent scar former, and minimizing the spillage of blood during surgery limits that scarring tendency. Second, in laparoscopic surgery, the tissues are handled very delicately and are constantly moistened with fluids, which also help prevent scar tissue from forming. Finally, with the absence of a large incision, there is less drying of the surfaces in the abdomen and less use of foreign materials, such as stitches and metal surgical clips, which all can be a cause for adhesions.

Therefore, because the surgeon is better able to see and identify the areas affected by endometriosis, because the entire abdomen can be seen, and because decreased tendencies toward the formation of adhesive disease are noted, the use of laparoscopy is the best surgical way to treat endometriosis. Simply put, the ability to do effective surgery depends on the surgeon's ability to see the problem and fix it. Laparoscopy best affords us that possibility. Of course, the bonus here for the patient is the overall decreased need for any prolonged recovery time. Patients who have laparoscopy are most often outpatient or "day surgery" cases, and they are able to return to most if not all normal activity within a few days.

What Is Laser Surgery vs. Excisional Surgery?

This is a matter mostly of semantics. In general, when someone talks about "laser surgery," they are talking about laparoscopy. Laparoscopy is the minimally invasive approach using a series of tiny incisions (less than a dime in size). Laparoscopic surgery became known as laser surgery because early in the development of this field, lasers were a common tool used for the surgery. We still use lasers today, as they can be extraordinarily helpful because of their accuracy and ability to cut tissue without causing bleeding.

Excisional surgery, on the other hand, refers to a specific technique of removing endometriosis completely by skinning or removing the entire area of endo down into the depths of the tissue. That is, instead of just cauterizing the area (the tissues are touched with a hot instrument) or vaporizing the endo (a laser is fired at the tissue, which eliminates a superficial layer of the abnormal area), the entire area of abnormality is actually removed using some type of cutting instrument. This can be done with scissors, a knife, or in our case a laser scalpel—i.e., "laser surgery."

Another advantage of excisional surgery is the ability to look microscopically at the removed tissues and document the presence of endometriosis. Although rare, other types of diseases can masquerade as endo, and at times it is critical to have tissue evidence of what is going on. Once I excised what I thought was endometriosis in a young women and later found out from the pathologist that the patient had ovarian cancer. Fortunately, because of that biopsy evidence, I was able to treat this very different disease successfully.

Excisional surgery also has the advantage of apparently long-lasting relief. In my clinic, 80 to 85 percent of women with mild to moderate disease achieved pain relief that lasted five to ten years or longer. Women with severe disease had symptom-free windows averaging three to five years and longer. This experience is consistent with clinics practicing excisional surgery around the United States and the world. Unfortunately, those clinics are somewhat few and far between, because surgeons who are experienced in this type of surgery are also rare. As the amount of data increases on this subject, increasing numbers of surgeons are willing to learn and master the skills necessary to provide more women with this alternative.

The Surgical Process

General anesthesia is the best choice for laparoscopic surgery. Through the years, my colleagues and I have experimented with using local anesthesia for this kind of surgery, but because of the position of the patient in surgery and for overall comfort, general anesthesia is the most common method used. The patient is tilted in a head-down position and carbon dioxide gas is used to inflate the abdomen—this is quite uncomfortable in an non-anaesthetized patient. This gas is evacuated at the end of the procedure but can be a source of pain during the procedure if the patient is awake. Also, manipulation of the internal organs can cause pain that is difficult to block without general anesthesia. In studies on using local anesthesia, "pain mapping" was attempted to find the sources of pelvic or abdominal pain in patients who were experiencing these symptoms. Although some of these studies were helpful in finding hidden endometriosis, most did not help us with this very difficult problem. Most of the patients involved then had to undergo another procedure to remove the areas that were found to be pain causers, many of which were already visible for excision without the pain mapping procedure.

Laparoscopy to remove endometriosis is done either at a hospital operating room or in a surgery center. Either of these two types of facilities is fine, because you rarely have to spend more than 24 hours in the center. I have had experience with both types of facilities and find that the surgery center is generally preferable because it typically focuses on the type of patient that I have. That is, most of my patients are not very sick, are having an elective procedure, and do not need high-tech advanced medical care. They just need a little "tender loving care."

Most often, a woman scheduled for laparoscopy enters the surgical facility in the morning. She'll not eat or drink after midnight on the night before the surgery. If there is any suspicion that there may be endometriosis involvement of the bowel, a bowel prep is also ordered for the day before surgery. This means the patient will be on a liquid diet and asked to drink a liquid that will cause a rapid transit of food through the gastrointestinal tract. She will go to the bathroom frequently for several hours after finishing the liquid. This clears the lower colon of solids and enables the surgeon to safely work on or around the bowel during the surgery. I routinely remove the appendix of women who have pelvic pain and endometriosis because this is a common site for recurrence of endo.

After the patient enters the center and speaks with the anesthesiologist and her surgeon, an intravenous (IV) line is started and she is transported into the operating room. Then she is moved to the operating room table and is given medicine through the IV that causes her to go to sleep. An hour or two later, she awakens in the recovery area. She might feel a bit confused in recovery, because she is still under the influence of the drugs used for anesthesia. From the recovery area, the patient either goes to extended recovery (like a hospital room where family/friends can come in to be with her) or goes home. The criteria for release to home are different from center to center, but it is important for the patient to feel comfortable with leaving and not feel rushed out of the facility.

During surgery, several tiny incisions are made in the patient's abdomen. The first incision is at or slightly under the belly button, and other incisions are added as necessary to accomplish the task at hand.

These incisions are all 1-centimeter (½ inch) or less in length. A tiny telescope is passed into the abdomen, and all abnormal areas are identified and marked for removal. The abnormal areas are removed down to the level of normal tissue below. Any scar tissue is also removed. Endometriomas (cysts of endometriosis usually found on or within the ovaries) are drained, and the internal portion of these cysts are removed. This technique has been shown to be better at limiting the recurrence of endometriosis and its associated problems.

Typical Recovery From Endometriosis Surgery

Most of my patients report that they are sore for the first couple of days, and they are able to resume all normal activities within seven to ten days. Patients are allowed to take care of themselves. They drive as soon as they feel comfortable doing so. This allows a patient to return to work easily within two weeks' time. If a patient's recovery is different from this, we feel obligated to investigate further. If a patient has had a bowel resection, the recovery can be a bit slower, but this is rare.

Hysterectomy as an Option for Endometriosis

There is no evidence that removal of the uterus, tubes, or ovaries does anything to eliminate endometriosis. However, a number of women do have other reasons for hysterectomy and also have endometriosis. Many of these women may need uterine removal but the endometriosis, if present, must be excised if the woman is to become pain-free and limit her need for future surgeries.

In other words, if a woman has abnormal uterine bleeding, this problem must be addressed. Abnormal bleeding is not a problem caused by endometriosis. In this case, if the patient also has endometriosis, then both of those problems must be addressed when surgery is performed. This may mean that a hysterectomy is needed, but not because of the endometriosis. The same is true with regard to ovaries. The ovaries may contain endo, but the disease can be removed and the ovaries preserved in the majority of cases. There is little evidence to support the suggestion that endometriosis will disappear in the absence of the hormonal activity produced by the ovaries.

If more extensive surgery such as hysterectomy is needed, this surgery can be performed laparoscopically with a recovery very similar to any other laparoscopic procedure. So, the recovery time, even with hysterectomy, does not change.

Endometriosis in Areas Other Than Pelvic Organs

In some cases, endometriosis may involve areas other than just the uterus, tubes, and ovaries. The appendix (which is part of the bowel) is the third most common area of occurrence of endo. For this reason, in women with pelvic pain, the appendix is always removed at the time of surgery. Studies by my colleagues and me have shown that most of these appendices that are removed are abnormal when studied by pathologists.

Since endometriosis can affect the bowel severely in some cases or the bladder in others, frequently surgeons from specialties other than gynecology may be involved in a woman's care. I believe that the ideal method of care is to have both general surgeons (for bowel care) and urologists (for bladder and urinary tract care) on the team and available to help the gynecologic surgeon who is directing the care of the women with endometriosis. Although it is uncommon to see disease of a severity that requires using these ancillary team members, it is very reassuring and efficient to have this capability available. A woman may or may not want to meet and discuss the plan with these other team members before surgery, but this consultation must be made available if that is the desire of the patient or her family.

Very rarely, we have encountered endometriosis in the area of the chest cavity, on or near the lungs or diaphragm. In this case, a thoracic surgeon is enlisted. Even in this situation, minimally invasive techniques can be used to correct the problem. Although the ability to deal with this problem is technically very difficult, this type of surgery is something that focused centers dealing with severe endometriosis can now do.

More on Adhesions

Adhesions can certainly be a very real problem after surgery. Adhesions are pieces of scar tissue that form on a surface or between the surfaces of organs in the abdomen. Areas that have been operated on and have any damage to their surfaces tend to stick together and form the scar-tissue bands called adhesions. These adhesions can be associated with pain and other problems, such as bowel obstruction, which can be very difficult to deal with.

During surgery, a number of steps should be taken to prevent adhesion formation after surgery. Careful handling of the tissues and carefully stopping any bleeding are key, as well as keeping the surfaces moist with special solutions that are known to prevent scarring. Prevention of adhesions is an active area of research. Adhesion barriers and adhesion prevention are significant areas of development that remain works in progress, but certainly laparoscopy lowers the risk of adhesion formation and makes this type of surgery important in reducing this potential for scarring.

The Right Doctor

As you can see, with all the specialized knowledge that is required to appropriately care of endometriosis, finding the right doctor is critical to successful treatment. It is also critical in making sure that you are not prescribed surgeries that are unnecessary for your case. And you want someone very skilled in endometriosis surgery to reduce post-surgical problems such as adhesions, to get you back on your feet quickly, and to give you a relatively pain-free post-surgery life.

The first thing any women who thinks she might have endometriosis (or any other problem, for that matter!) must do is to find out as much about the disease as she can. First, talk to your friends and others who have had similar experiences. They can provide amazing information and support that you wouldn't imagine. Second, talk to your physician or practitioner. This may be helpful or confusing, but it is essential to know what knowledge your day-to-day caregiver has and how he or she can help you. Third, be sure to do your own research in books, on the Internet, and through available organizations. Today, the Internet is the most fertile ground for up-to-the-minute research and can provide more information quickly than any other resource. With all this information in hand, you can then try to find the right doctor for you.

During this selection process, don't be afraid to ask questions and demand answers to those questions until you are satisfied with the information provided. Check the surgeon's background. Ask if the doctor has statistics regarding success or failure of treatment. Specifically with surgeons, ask how often they treat endometriosis surgically and whether they have a team to treat more advanced disease. Are they laparoscopic surgeons, and, if so, how often have they needed to change to a large incision to finish the job? This last question is called the "rate of conversion" and may be one of the most important pieces of information to know when selecting a surgeon.

Without question, it is preferable to use a clinic that specializes in or emphasizes endometriosis. Very few, if any, general obstetricians/gynecologists (OB/GYNs) are the best choice for endometriosis because of lack of experience with this difficult disorder. They may be great OB/GYNs, but treatment for a disease like endometriosis benefits greatly from a lot of experience with the specific disease. Although this is a good place to start, make sure that you are satisfied with the answers to those critical questions.

I believe that endometriosis can be an extremely difficult medical case. The surgical aspect of endo care is probably the most complex part of the overall care, but it is the most critical in many respects. It is essential that the surgical component of your care be under the control of surgeons with experience and surgical teams with multi-specialty capacities. This can allow more efficient, effective care for women with endometriosis, who have been rather uniformly under-served up to this time. In addition to this elite group of surgeons, pain management specialists as well as psychotherapists and holistic practitioners should be brought onto the team to round out the options for these difficult cases.

CHAPTER FIVE ∾

Pain Management

Pain management could fill volumes of books and still leave subjects not discussed. I've already said that pain is the most significant symptom associated with endometriosis, so pain must be dealt with. First, some common questions on this subject.

How Does Endometriosis Cause Pain?

I knew that sooner or later this would come up, and, to be very honest, no one really knows. I'll give you some ideas that might be an explanation, but understand that none of this is known fact. One thing that we are sure of is that endometriosis is an irritating force that causes the body to be inflamed where the endometriosis is growing. Anything that causes inflammation can cause pain. Tissues of the body that are inflamed release various chemicals called prostaglandins, substance P, kallikreins, and other agents, and somehow these chemicals cause pain. That's a very sketchy description of what is an extremely complicated process, but this is one fairly well understood "pain pathway." This is why one type of drug therapies is intended to decrease the amount of chemical irritants being produced. Also, this inflammation/irritation can cause scarring, and scarring can in turn cause pain. There are multiple other theoretical pain pathways. For example, swelling can also produce pain. Various tissues in the body, such as the ovaries, can swell or enlarge due to the growth of endometriosis from within (endometrioma), or tissue may swell as a reaction to inflammation. There can be direct pain where an area of the body is inflamed and pain whenever these areas are disturbed or touched.

For example, if the space at the very back of the vagina or the utero-sacral ligaments are affected by endometriosis, then intercourse logically would cause pain (dyspareunia) just from the direct contact with the inflamed tissue. At the same time, endo in this area could cause pain with bowel movements. Stool is solid in this area of the colon and can further irritate the inflamed tissue as it passes through, causing painful bowel movements (dyschezia). Through these and other, less well understood means, endometriosis can cause severe, chronic, and debilitating pain that can significantly affect women's lives. The constancy of the pain may be one of the worst problems (more on that later).

If I Have Severe Pain, Am I Untreatable or a Hopeless Case?

Interestingly, the level of pain does not necessarily correspond to the severity of the disease. Some patients with very severe endometriosis have severe symptoms, and some have very little in the way of pain. At the same time, some women with a very small amount of disease have severe symptoms. This can be very confusing to a woman and her doctor, particularly if that doctor has little experience with or understanding of endometriosis. Unfortunately, some women with endometriosis are therefore labeled as delusional and treated as if they have psychiatric problems or not taken seriously when severe disease is present due to lack of severe symptoms. This is one of the most difficult problems with this disease.

A doctor's ability to listen to you and to communicate clearly is extremely important for you as an endometriosis patient. A team approach can be helpful with problems that can range from straightforward excision to more difficult, complex infertility with significant pain and psychosocial overtones. Occasionally, a combination approach is necessary, but virtually all patients with pain that is related to endometriosis are able to recover completely.

If the Pain Goes Away, Will it Come Back?

This is a difficult question, as it really depends on your particular case. Generally speaking, there is no known cure for endometriosis, and so there is no guarantee that successful treatment will give you permanent relief of symptoms or pain. However, many women are able to achieve lasting (years) relief when appropriate therapies are used. I discuss in detail what these therapies may be in this and other chapters. Statistics are available on these results, but in my opinion, no data reliably predicts when or if the pain will return. Some data on surgical excision speaks to this question, but there is no data on endo treatment in general.

What Causes Pain In General?

This is the $64,000 question. The sequence goes something like this. First, there is an injury or irritation of tissue somewhere in the body either from a mechanical (cutting, crushing, burning, freezing, stretching) or a chemical source (acid, prostaglandins, substance P). The stimulus of the injury/irritation is transmitted by nerve impulses to the spinal cord, which carries this signal to the brain. The brain perceives the signal as pain. Therefore, most treatments for pain revolve around doing something to change this chain of events.

Methods of Treating Pain

Enough of the anatomy lessons, let's get down to the methods that are currently being used to treat people with pain. I'll take this step by step, and although I can't include everything, hopefully you'll have a good idea of what is available and what I've found that works on the majority of patients.

Obviously, the first goal would be to remove or reduce the stimulus causing the pain. That means eliminating the endometriosis, if possible. The only way I know of to accomplish this task is surgical removal of the disease. Of course, you have to recognize the disease so it can be removed and, as in cancer, the surgeon wants to completely remove the disease. As discussed in Chapter Four, these goals can be very difficult. However, in my experience, the best long-lasting pain relief to date is achieved through surgical removal of the endometriosis.

Many drugs for eliminating endometriosis have been tried, but none have succeeded. However, some of these treatments have been successful in stopping or altering the stimulus for pain and, thereby, eliminating or altering the transmission of the pain signal to the brain. For example, the irritation/inflammation stimulus can be improved by decreasing the hormone activity in tissues that are hormonally responsive (uterus, fallopian tubes, ovaries, and surrounding structures). Using drugs like Lupron or Danazol causes this to happen by creating a menopause-like state where hormone activity is nil. Birth control pills or progestogenic drugs (Depo-Provera, Provera, Norlutate, and others) also cause a decrease in hormone activity and, at least in some cases, a decrease in pain. These medications can significantly reduce pain in a large number of people, but the pain relief only lasts for the amount of time you're taking the medicine. If you stop taking the medicine, your symptoms will likely recur within a very short time. The other problem with this type of medication is that, in general, hormonal manipulation like this does not allow you to become pregnant and some women are actively seeking pregnancy.

Other types of drugs that seek to eliminate the initial stimulus try to counteract the biochemical actions that cause the pain stimulus. The drugs in this family are called the non-steroidal anti-inflammatory drugs, or NSAIDs. NSAIDS are generally prostaglandin inhibitors, which seek to reduce the amount of prostaglandins (biochemical "bad guys") painful areas and thereby decrease that initial pain stimulus. Aspirin, Advil, Aleve, Anaprox, Vioxx, Bextra, and Celebrex are examples of these drugs. Some are available over the counter, and others must be obtained by prescription from a doctor. All have been helpful at reducing pain, but the pain relief is limited to the time that the drug is taken plus a few hours after. Side effects are fairly limited but must be considered. Most people, unfortunately, live by the philosophy that if a little medicine is good then a lot will be better. Liver problems and high blood pressure can develop in some people taking these drugs.

Many of these drugs have been shown to irritate the stomach and are not recommended in people with stomach ulcers or other stomach problems. So even though these medications are generally safe and available without a prescription, be sure to follow package instructions and, most importantly, if pain persists, check with your doctor about what to do next. Pain is not a symptom to be ignored—its source should be carefully identified.

Some medicines work to relieve pain at the other end of the pain reaction. These drugs are in the general area of opioids (narcotics), and they distort the perception in the brain of the painful stimulus. Morphine, Codeine, Lortab, Vicodan, Percocet, Dilaudid, Oxycontin, and Demerol are all medicines that are limited to prescription use. All have a significant risk of addiction if used for prolonged lengths of time. I rarely prescribe these drugs except in the immediate post-surgical time period for the pain associated with surgery. Otherwise, I don't believe that there is a primary place for them unless all other alternatives have been exhausted. Obviously, women of reproductive age should not be taking these drugs while attempting pregnancy. The opioids all produce a euphoric ("high") feeling, which can be appropriate if you're having a severe level of pain but can be difficult if you need to be functional and able to care for yourself.

The opiates also can produce some other side effects. There is an overall depressant effect on both bowel and bladder performance.

Constipation and inability to urinate normally can be seen with these medicines. There is also a risk of slowing the breathing, so people who have any lung or other respiratory problems should be very careful when using these medications. The possibility of becoming addicted to these drugs must be considered at all times and, therefore, careful management under the watchful eye of your doctor is a requirement. In short, opiates are good for short-term use under a doctor's management.

Other drugs that work in a similar fashion by decreasing anxiety (Xanax, Valium, Phenergan) or relaxing your muscles can have a positive effect on pain reduction by putting you more at ease and thereby increasing your pain threshold. These drugs would be called psychotropic agents. Another class of medicines in this category is the antidepressant medicines, from classic antidepressants such as Elavil to the more recent additions such as Prozac and Serafem. Usually, these drugs are used in conjunction with other medications or therapies to produce a lasting, long-term relief. Side effects from most of these drugs are minimal, limited, and reversible. Also, there may be a therapeutic advantage to using antidepressants for chronic pain because depression is routinely found in people having to deal with chronic pain.

Another class of drugs used in pain relief decreases the overall irritability of the nervous system. Many of these drugs are also used as anti-seizure medications. Neurontin, Tegretol, and phenobarbital have been used with success to treat chronic pain and related symptoms. These drugs are frequently used in addition to or in conjunction with other medications to successfully reduce the painful stimuli. Side effects may be a factor, and some of the medicines require ongoing testing for liver problems and blood clotting factors as well as medical monitoring for general well-being. These drugs seem to be evolving into the most interesting class of medical therapies for managing pain because of their inherent safety and lack of addictive potential.

If drug treatment or surgical interventions have failed, there are still options for you. If you have a sore spot or a "trigger point" where pain can be elicited by touching or pushing on a point, then trigger point injections can be attempted. In this procedure, a local anesthetic (xylocaine, novocaine, marcaine) can be injected into the trigger point area along with, at times, a steroid solution (cortisone), which further reduces inflammation. In some cases, this treatment eliminates or significantly reduces pain. If trigger point injections are successful, they may last for weeks, months or indefinitely. Obviously, if successful, the injections can be repeated at whatever interval seems necessary in each individual. Most often this type of treatment is administered by a physician who specializes in pain therapy. Most of these doctors are trained as anesthesiologists, physiatrists (physical medicine and rehabilitation), or orthopedists, and many get further training in pain medicine. Some gynecologists have obtained training in this type of medicine, but more often, we just develop a relationship with a pain specialist who meets the needs of our patients and work together to solve a patient's problems.

Another type of "nerve block" may also be appropriate for patients with pelvic pain. This block is made close to the spinal cord and requires the skill to locate and isolate the nerves to be blocked. The procedure can be performed under no anesthesia but frequently may require x-ray (fluoroscopy) guidance. For these blocks, a needle is passed into the space just outside the spinal cord, and local anesthetic is injected into this area. The anesthetic can "block" the entire area covered by a particular nerve and is quite effective, but the amount of time that it lasts can vary depending on a number of variables. This procedure is also called an epidural block and is commonly used during labor and delivery at childbirth.

Again, this procedure must be done only by doctors who have expertise in this area. Various types of blocks are available, and different anesthetics can be used to achieve a result that is productive for each individual. Of course, nothing has been done to the source of the pain, but if symptoms are relieved in these difficult situations, success is achieved. Sometimes, if necessary, a tiny flexible telescope can be inserted into the epidural space around the spinal cord, and the area can be inspected to see if there is scarring around a nerve or a space that could be treated and allow pain relief.

In general, nerve blocks can be either therapeutic or diagnostic. Sometimes a nerve block can be used to isolate or find the source of a person's pain. Different types of anesthetics can be used to cause a temporary block or a more permanent one. A permanent block can give more prolonged relief of pain that has been first isolated by using a short-acting anesthetic. Blockade of a nerve bundle is called a sympathetic block and is commonly used in most pain clinics. For a sympathetic block, an x-ray is frequently used to isolate an area and then a block using a temporary anesthetic is placed. After the patient's response to the temporary agent is assessed, a permanent agent or stimulator may be used to achieve long-term pain control.

A relatively new treatment for people with chronic pain disorders involves stimulation of the nerves involved in the pain. This procedure is based on the spinal gate theory. In this theory, pain stimuli are seen entering the spinal cord through a gate. The gate is only wide enough to allow a few nerve impulses to get through. According to the theory, bombarding the area with electrical impulses from a generator carried by the patient fills the gate with information so the pain information is unable pass through. Thus, the patient's pain is relieved.

These stimulators were originally used only externally and required no surgery. Now spinal stimulators are placed close to or on the spine or nerve in question, and an internal generator that can be controlled externally is inserted under the skin. The external controls allow modulation or fine tuning of the stimulator until optimal pain relief is achieved. This type of placement requires specific training and expertise and should only be used if your condition is properly evaluated and you are well-informed about the procedure's pros and cons.

Physical therapy is frequently used in association with medical or surgical therapy to improve painful symptoms. Massage, stretching, ultrasound, electrical stimulation, hydrotherapy, hot packs, cold packs, and various exercise regimens can be used effectively to treat pain and improve your response after medical or surgical treatment. These treatments may improve swelling and increase motion in an area, which can aid both short-term and long-term recovery.

As you can see, the management of pain has become highly technically oriented. Interestingly, though, many pain management specialists have begun to use ancient means of controlling pain. Acupuncture, which dates back at least several hundred years, is used effectively by practitioners across the United States. The methods of diagnosis used in acupuncture are based on the theory that the function of the internal organ, the flow of blood and lymph, and the emotional state of an individual have specific observable influences in their external or visible appearance. The selection of the needles and point application of these needles are based on this pattern of physical findings. I have had several patients who were successful with this mode of treatment, which has a basis in ancient Asian culture. Interestingly, this same culture has produced some herbal remedies that have become the mainstay of current drug treatments (opium/morphine).

Behavioral medicine also plays a significant role in the treatment of women with pain related to endometriosis. Originally, this discipline was devoted to those diseases caused by or made worse by stress. Of course, more and more practitioners are willing to admit that stress and other psychosocial influences play a significant role in the diseases and day-to-day lives of their patients. Cognitive and behavioral therapies have been developed to address this need. These therapies involve learning and applying behavioral skills that can help you deal with stress and other influences that cause problems. Biofeedback, relaxation techniques, diary keeping, pacing activities, and psychotherapy are all part of this treatment. Behavioral medicine can be extremely helpful for some people, especially when paired with effective medical and surgical solutions.

Pain assumed to be related to or caused by endometriosis can be due to other causes. For example, bowel problems such as irritable bowel syndrome (IBS) or inflammatory bowel disease (IBD, Crohn's disease, regional enteritis), diverticular disease, appendicitis, kidney stones, interstitial cystitis (IC), and many other problems can cause abdominal or pelvic pain similar to that caused by endometriosis. For this reason, your doctor should thoroughly examine you, ask questions about your medical history, and counsel you about these problems. Your doctor should also rule out bowel disorders and kidney or bladder disease before assuming your pain is from endometriosis. In turn, keep in mind that the presence of endometriosis does not exclude the presence of any of these problems either. Common co-conspirators with endometriosis are IBS, IC, and appendix problems. Although some of these things can be treated during endometriosis surgery, others must be managed in a completely different manner and require a totally separate drug regimen that does not always mesh with typical endo therapy.

As you can see by the wandering nature of this chapter, pain management can be a daunting task for the patient and her medical practitioner. Because many patients with endometriosis experience no symptoms, the rationale for treatment is variable and not always based on pure science. If we had a cure for endometriosis, I would think that pain management would be a rather simple proposition and could easily be handled by eradication of the disease. However, in this complicated scenario where the treatment itself (surgery) can cause adhesions and, therefore, pain, it can be difficult to decide on and apply these treatments. At this time, surgery seems to be my best tool. However, this tool is no good without the safety net of medical therapies and pain management to wage war against the formidable enemy of endometriosis.

What Are Pain Management Clinics?

Wherever you find "medical malls" where medical offices group together, you'll almost always find, amidst the dentists and neurologists and mammography centers, something called a pain management clinic.

The phrase pain management was first used in medical literature by Dr. Joseph Bianca in 1953. Pain management clinics are designed to help patients with any kind of pain that stems from any source. Here you can receive help for headaches, neck aches, backaches, and much more.

The goal of most pain management clinics is to break the cycle of pain. They are interested in working with you on as long a term basis as you need to alleviate or eliminate pain. How successful your treatment is, of course, depends on the source of your pain and how much it can be alleviated.

Northeast Pain Consultation and Management, which opened in 1992, was the first freestanding pain management clinic in New Hampshire. According to its administrator, Monica Haley, pain management clinics can have several different approaches:

- Behavioral modification, where only the psychological component of pain is dealt with
- Pain blocking, which is strictly medical intervention to block the pain

• A hybrid clinic, where medical management and counseling as well as physical therapy and perhaps some complementary medical approaches are practiced

Most clinics, Haley says, only take referrals from your primary care physician. Some take self-referrals. And some insurance providers cover the cost of pain management clinic visits.

To be sure you are dealing with a reputable clinic, Haley advises that you:

• Check the credentials of the clinic's practitioners
• Always be sure there is a board-certified physician associated with the clinic
• Make sure that the approach they use is appropriate for your case
• Be sure you have a good patient/doctor fit

The work of a pain management clinic can be quite extensive and comprehensive. Northeast asks new patients to complete and mail back a preliminary four-page questionnaire before their first visit. The clinic also requires your complete medical records to review ahead of time. Any diagnostic tests that you have had—ultrasounds, x-rays, etc.—can be brought with you to the appointment. The initial visit takes two hours, including a half hour with the administrator going through your paper-work, a half hour with a nurse, and an hour with the doctor. Don't worry about telling too many details; by the time you are done with your first visit, the pain management clinic staff will have left no stone unturned!

What Can I Do on My Own for General Pain Relief?

When you're trying to find pain relief, keep these simple things in mind:

- Find ways to relax and relieve pain before bed. Pain affects how you sleep, and getting a good night's rest affects how much pain you feel. Try listening to relaxing music, using aromatherapy treatments such as a lavender pillow near your bed, or taking a warm bath or shower—anything you find relaxing that might ultimately help you sleep.

- Make notes of your pain experiences. Record pain levels in the morning, midday, and at night. Do this for a month or more and look for patterns. Does your pain get worse when you're under stress? When you don't get enough sleep or overdo exercise? Use those patterns to try to get the pain in check before it happens or gets too intense.

- Don't use alcohol to relieve pain. It just doesn't work over the longterm. If you drink one glass of wine or a cold beer in the evening as part of your relaxation routine, fine; but do not consume more alcohol to relieve pain symptoms. Alcohol, of course, can become addicting, and it ultimately causes sleep disturbance, which will only work against you.

- Keep a list of some things to do for pain as it worsens. Be prepared in advance, since pain can cause you to not think as clearly. Try listing your options in the order of how much each activity helps in regard to the intensity or longevity of the pain episode.

Severe chronic pain affects one in ten Americans, according to the National Chronic Pain Outreach Association (www.chronicpain.org). This information clearinghouse on pain management and research also lists support groups around the country for anyone dealing with chronic pain.

You can find a list of pain management clinics throughout the country at www.painlinks.org.

A PERSONAL STORY

Marybeth

Now 46, Marybeth started her period when she was 10 years old. Even then she suffered badly each month, starting mostly with uterine cramps. Then the pain spread to include backaches and side aches, and she would bloat as much as an extra eleven pounds.

Marybeth saw her family doctor regularly, but pre-menstrual syndrome wasn't much talked about then. In fact, when she tried to get help for her symptoms, the doctor asked her, "What is this problem you have with accepting being a woman?" As a kid, she recalls, she just didn't know what to make of it all.

Marybeth saw a gynecologist for the first time in 1970, when she was thirteen. He didn't do anything for her symptoms. Later, when she was a freshman in college, she had a D&C. Not only was it very painful, but it didn't help relieve her symptoms. However, the doctor who performed the surgery was the first to bring up endometriosis. He told her that having a baby would cure it.

Her doctor before that had told her that being on the pill would cure her problems. It did help some with the pain symptoms, but the pill's side effects made her very ill.

Marybeth then saw a fertility specialist, who found that she had a double uterus. By then, a new study had come out about so-called DES daughters. DES (diethyl-stilbestrol) was a common drug administered to women in the 1950s and 1960s to prevent miscarriage. A double uterus was discovered to be common in daughters of women who took DES.

By now, Marybeth was suffering with pain an entire week out of each month, with no solution in sight. "I even tried alcohol," she admits, "but I couldn't drink enough to kill the pain without being totally incoherent." Her dysmenorrhea—irregular menstrual cycles—and her pain inhibited every activity she tried to participate in, every event or family gathering she tried to attend, every class, even work.

Around 1978, Marybeth began to dabble in alternative medicine. She heard about a nutrition clinic presented by a dentist; she attended in an attempt to gain any information she could about healthful eating habits. The dentist added a bit more inspiration than simply good eating—he offered the message, "your body is your best doctor, don't let anyone lessen your pain." This advice would help her through years of trying to gain control of her health.

In the early 1980s, Marybeth was ready to start a family. She started seeing a fertility specialist, who told her she should not wait to have a child. In 1982, she had her first child with the help of doctors from the maternal high-risk group at the local university. She breastfed for thirteen months, so for almost two years she didn't have enough of a menstrual cycle to know what might be going on with her endometriosis. She got pregnant again, but this time miscarried at twenty weeks.

"When I started my periods regularly again," Marybeth recalls, "I went right back to the same endometriosis issues, just as bad as before." For the next six years—when she got pregnant again—she was sick quite a bit.

After Marybeth had her second child, the endometriosis again went back to business as usual. Her doctor recommended a hysterectomy. She resisted until age 36, but finally they agreed to the surgery. However, the surgery was postponed because of Marybeth's mother's illness and subsequent death. Her experience with her mother's illness gave her some issues of trust with hospitals that would make Marybeth hold off three years before rescheduling her hysterectomy. At age 39, she finally had the surgery.

"This has made a huge difference," Marybeth says with enormous relief. "My whole life, until I was 39 years old, was spent having to accomplish everything in three weeks out of each month."

Does Marybeth have advice for other women? You bet. First, Marybeth wishes she had started focusing on nutrition when she was ten instead of in her twenties. "This is a huge thing that people should not ignore," she says.

She also has words of wisdom for how women handle their own health and work with the medical community. "You have to go beyond proactive," she says, "and be demanding. Demand that someone fix your suffering—don't let them blow you off."

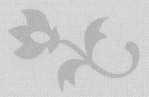

CHAPTER SIX ∾

Endometriosis Plus
Related Health Concerns

As the amount of endometriosis-centered research increases, so does the list of other health issues that doctors feel are related to this disease. This may sound dire—as if you're going to have to deal with a bunch of problems, rather than one, but on an upbeat note, the overlapping nature of health conditions that co-exist with endo may lead to a more complete understanding of this complex disease. In other words, knowing that endometriosis may exist in concert with other illnesses is actually a step in the right direction.

Nevertheless, this positive point-of-view doesn't dismiss the fact that women with endometriosis will likely find their health further compromised by other opportunistic symptoms. This chapter spotlights the most common conditions that accompany endometriosis.

Although a woman dealing with endometriosis would certainly rather not deal with other health issues at the same time, ignoring these issues is worse than facing them head on. Knowing that other health problems can co-exist with endo may lead to better diagnosis and treatment and improved quality of life. And as always with endometriosis, individual experience with the range of health conditions related to endo can range from minimal to disabling. As you read this chapter, perhaps you will gather some clues to help you better understand the complexities of endo. And you may even help your doctor help you, since you may not have thought to mention some of these things to your health care team.

Autoimmune (Dis)Connection?

Beginning in 1980, Endometriosis Association research demonstrated links between endometriosis, allergies, and other evidence of problems with the immune system. This correlation led to further research on which diseases were more prevalent in women with endometriosis.

Teams of researchers from the Endometriosis Association in Milwaukee, the National Institute of Child Health and Human Development, and the School of Public Health and Health Services at George Washington University distributed and analyzed a survey of 3,680 women with endometriosis. They published their findings in the October 2002 issue of the Human Reproduction medical journal.

They found:

- Twenty percent had more than one other disease.
- Up to 31 percent of those with co-existing diseases had

been diagnosed with either fibromyalgia, which is twice as common among women with endometriosis as among the general female population, or chronic fatigue syndrome, which is more than a hundred times as likely. Some of these women also had other autoimmune or endocrine diseases.

• Autoimmune inflammatory diseases—such as systemic lupus erythematosus, Sjögren's syndrome, rheumatoid arthritis, and multiple sclerosis—occurred more frequently among women with endometriosis.

• Hypothyroidism was seven times more common.

• Allergic conditions such as asthma and eczema were significantly higher. Twelve percent of women with endometriosis had asthma, compared to 5 percent of women without endo. Among women with endometriosis plus an endocrine disease, 72 percent had allergies; and among women with endometriosis plus fibromyalgia or chronic fatigue syndrome, the figure rose to 88 percent.

• Sixty-one percent of endometriosis sufferers had allergies, compared to 18 percent of the general U.S. population.

• Two-thirds of women with endo reported that they had family members with diagnosed or suspected endometriosis, confirming research that suggests there is a familial tendency.

"These findings suggest a strong association between endometriosis and autoimmune disorders," said Ninet Sinaii, the study's lead investigator from the National Institute of Child Health and Human Development, in the report. "Health care professionals may need to consider these disorders when evaluating their patients for endometriosis."

Mary Lou Ballweg, president of the Endometriosis Association and co-investigator of the study, said, "It is gratifying that the bigger picture of endometriosis as a serious immune and endocrine disease is finally coming to light. From our earliest research we were aware of the immune dysfunction common in women with endometriosis and their families. These important findings should spur more research."

These findings are also in concert with the similarities between endometriosis and cancer. It is certainly well known in the medical community that there is an association with immune system problems and malignant diseases. That there seems to be a similar alliance with endometriosis certainly is not surprising. I don't mean that endometriosis is a cancer, but these two diseases do share some common ground.

Attention All Women!

Doctors don't understand why, but about 75 percent of autoimmune diseases occur in women. There are many types of autoimmune diseases, but they all stem from the body's immune system mistakenly attacking healthy cells or tissues. Because certain autoimmune illnesses appear more frequently after menopause, others suddenly improve during pregnancy, and still others get worse during pregnancy, researchers and physicians believe hormones play a role in the problem.

Although individual autoimmune diseases are not very common, with the exception of thyroid disease, diabetes, and systemic lupus erythematosus (SLE), as a category of disease, they represent the fourth-largest cause of disability among women in the United States. In other words, although small numbers of women suffer from specific diseases, when you take all of the autoimmune diseases together, they comprise a huge problem for women—something on the level of heart disease and cancers.

Doctors divide these diseases into two major categories, based on two factors that contribute to the presence of autoimmune diseases: genetics and environment. Virtually every autoimmune disease combines these two culprits.

In terms of genetics, autoimmune diseases tend to run in families. If one person in a family has an autoimmune disease, it is likely that another family member will have one too, though, ironically, it probably won't be the same condition. No one understands why this is, although it is certainly something researchers are studying.

Likewise, research is shedding light on genetic as well as hormonal and environmental risk factors that contribute to the causes of these diseases.

According to the American Autoimmune Related Diseases Association, Inc., "Autoimmune diseases remain among the most poorly understood and poorly recognized of any category of illnesses. Individual diseases range from the benign to the severe. Symptoms vary widely, notably from one illness to another, but even within the same disease. And because the diseases affect multiple body systems, their symptoms are often misleading, which hinders accurate diagnosis."

What Is an Autoimmune Disease?

The immune system is normally the body's first line of defense against infection and other foreign "invaders." At the heart of the system is the ability to recognize and respond to substances called antigens, whether they are infectious agents or part of the body (self-antigens), as is the case with endometrial lesions.

A healthy immune system generates ten million antibody proteins every hour to counteract pathogens such as viruses, fungi, parasites, or rogue cells. When a person has an autoimmune disease, the immune system mistakenly targets the cells, tissues, and organs of a person's own body as it would a pathogen.

There is a system built into all of the cells in the body called the major histocompatibility complex (MHC) that marks the cells in your body as "you." Any cell that does not have your markings raises the guard of your immune system.

MHC molecules are important components of the immune response. They allow cells that have been invaded by an infectious organism to be detected by cells of the immune system called T-lymphocytes, also known as T-cells. The MHC molecules do this by presenting fragments of proteins (peptides) belonging to the invader on the surface of the infected cell. The T-cell recognizes the foreign peptide attached to the MHC molecule and binds to it. This stimulates the T-cell to either destroy or cure the infected cell. In uninfected healthy cells, the MHC molecule presents peptides from its own cell (self-peptides), to which T-cells do not normally react. However, if the immune mechanism malfunctions and T-cells react against self-peptides, an autoimmune disease arises.

Autoimmune Disorders

Because the evidence is strong that many autoimmune conditions may individually or collectively co-exist with endometriosis (which could prove to be an autoimmune condition itself, given time and research), the next section describes those that are most likely to further challenge your health and diagnosis. As you'll see, many of these related health problems include symptoms that overlap with not only endometriosis but also each other, adding complexity to the process of trying to understand an already complicated disease.

Autoimmune Symptoms

Symptoms common to many autoimmune diseases generally include the following:

> *Fatigue*: Anxious, uncomfortable fatigue related to lack of sleep or a disruption of the energy production mechanism in cells, either from lack of oxygen, increased toxicity, infections or a malfunction of the mitochondria.

Gastrointestinal problems: Ranging from gas, bloating, cramps, diarrhea, and constipation to hiatal hernia, irritable bowel syndrome, and Crohn's disease.

Fibromyalgia: Often diagnosed as a separate condition, fibromyalgia is basically a symptom of autoimmune disease. Fibromyalgia itself is diagnosed from the presence of pain in at least 11 of 18 specific sites on the body.

Candida yeast infections: As described in Chapter One, Candida is an infection caused by a common yeast-like fungus, Candida albicans. This fungus normally abounds in the mouth, throat, vagina, and intestines in balance with other bacteria and yeasts in the body. It becomes problematic if a pH imbalance causes the fungus to multiply, creating long branches of yeast cells known as candidiasis.

Allergies

People with allergies have a hyper-vigilant immune system. Exposure to what is normally a harmless substance, such as pollen, causes the immune system to react as if the substance (allergen) is a harmful invader. The body starts to produce a specific type of antibody called IgE to fight the allergen, which attaches to a type of blood cell called a mast cell. Mast cells are plentiful in the airways and in the gastro-intestinal tract, where allergens tend to enter the body. The mast cells release a variety of chemicals including histamine, which causes most of the symptoms of an allergy. If the allergen is in the air, the allergic reaction will occur in the eyes, nose, and lungs. If the allergen is ingested, the allergic reaction will occur in the mouth, stomach, and intestines. Sometimes enough chemicals are released from the mast cells to cause a reaction throughout the body, such as hives, decreased blood pressure, shock, or loss of consciousness. A severe reaction is called anaphylaxis and may be life-threatening.

Allergy symptoms can be categorized as mild, moderate, or severe (anaphylactic). Mild reactions include those symptoms that affect a specific area of the body, such as a rash or hives, itchy and watery eyes, and some congestion. Mild reactions do not spread to other parts of the body.

Moderate reactions include symptoms that spread to other parts of the body. These may include itchiness or difficulty in breathing.

A severe reaction (anaphylaxis) is a life-threatening emergency in which the body's response to the allergen is sudden and affects the whole body. It may begin with the sudden onset of itching of the eyes or face and within minutes progress to more serious symptoms, including varying degrees of swelling as in hives (if the airways or throat are involved in the swelling, this could result in difficulty swallowing and breathing), abdominal pain, cramps, vomiting, and diarrhea. Mental confusion or dizziness may also be symptoms, since anaphylaxis causes a quick drop in blood pressure.

A blood test called the "Food Antibody Assessment IgE & IgG" can identify foods that cause allergic reactions.

Autoimmune Thyroid Diseases

Hashimoto's thyroiditis and Graves' disease result from immune system destruction or stimulation of thyroid tissue. Symptoms of low (hypo-) or overactive (hyper-) thyroid function are nonspecific and can develop slowly or suddenly. These symptoms include fatigue, moderate weight gain, depression, cold or heat intolerance, weakness, dry skin and brittle hair, and infertility. Left untreated, thyroid disorder can elevate cholesterol and triglyceride levels, leading to hardening of the arteries. Hashimoto's thyroiditis, also referred to as autoimmune thyroiditis or chronic lymphocytic thyroiditis, is a chronic inflammatory disease of the glands caused by an autoimmune reaction to proteins in the thyroid. Antibodies bind to the thyroid and prevent it from producing the right balance of the thyroid hormones L-triiodothyronine (T3) and L-thyroxine (T4). Approximately 25 percent of patients with Hashimoto's may develop pernicious anemia, diabetes, adrenal insufficiency, or other autoimmune diseases.

Graves' disease can eventually destroy the thyroid, resulting in hypo-thyroidism. More commonly, the person has an enlarged thyroid gland even when thyroid function tests are normal or mildly abnormal. The source of Graves' disease and the method by which it causes problems for the thyroid gland is not well understood, but it is basically an in-flammatory process of questionable source. Apparently, diet and heredity are contributors but little is known to support absolute explanations for the disease.

Candidiasis

The long list of symptoms of candidiasis includes constipation, diarrhea, colitis, abdominal pain, headaches, bad breath, rectal itching, mood swings, memory loss, facial numbness, night sweats, clogged sinuses, white spots on the tongue and mouth (thrush), pre-menstrual syndrome (PMS), extreme fatigue, vaginitis, urinary tract infections, arthritis, depression, heartburn, sore throat, hyperthyroidism, and adrenal problems. In severe cases, Candida can travel through the bloodstream and invade other organ systems, causing a type of blood poisoning called Candida septicemia.

Candidiasis is frequently evident in people with compromised immune systems and is often accompanied by food and environmental allergies. Prolonged or frequent antibiotic use, which damages the "friendly" bacteria that control Candida, allowing it to multiply, is another contributing factor.

Many women with gastrointestinal symptoms have found relief from treatment of candidiasis, including nutritional strategies and strengthening their immune systems. See Chapter Seven for immune-building strategies and Chapter Eight for information on nutritional support.

Chronic Fatigue Syndrome

A diagnosis of chronic fatigue syndrome is based on the following criteria from the U.S. Centers for Disease Control and Prevention (CDC): an unexplained, persistent, relapsing chronic fatigue that has not been of long duration, is not reduced by adequate rest, and affects quality of life.

According to the CDC, four or more of the following symptoms must be present along with the presence of severe fatigue. These symptoms persist or recur during six or more consecutive months and were not present before the onset of the severe chronic fatigue:

- Headaches of a new type, pattern, or severity
- Muscle pains (multi-joint pain without swelling or redness)
- Malaise after physical exertion that lasts more than twenty-four hours
- Sore throat
- Substantial impairment in short-term memory or concentration
- Tender lymph nodes
- Unrefreshing sleep

Eczema (Atopic Dermatitis)

Eczema is a common allergic reaction often affecting the face, elbows, and knees. This red, scaly, itchy rash is typically seen in young infants but can occur later in life in individuals with personal or family histories of asthma or allergic rhinitis (hay fever). In adults, the patches are usually dry, red to brownish-gray, and may be scaly or thickened. The disease does not always follow the usual pattern and may appear on the palms, backs of the hands and fingers, or on the feet, where crusting, oozing, thickened areas may last for years. The itching may be intense, almost unbearable, and may be most noticeable at night. Some patients scratch the skin until it bleeds and crusts. When this occurs, the skin can get infected.

Common triggers include overheating or sweating and contact with irritants such as wool, pets, or soaps. Emotional stress can also cause a flare-up. Rarely, certain foods can trigger eczema.

Fibromyalgia Syndrome

FMS (fibromyalgia syndrome) is a widespread musculoskeletal pain and fatigue disorder. The cause is still unknown. Fibromyalgia means pain in the fibrous tissues in the body: muscles, ligaments, and tendons. It typically mimics a yeast infection but without the typical discharge. Intense PMS and cramping are common, and all symptoms of fibromyalgia are worse pre-menstrually.

Most patients with fibromyalgia say that they ache all over. Their muscles may feel like they have been pulled or overworked. Sometimes the muscles twitch and at other times they burn. Here's an overview of symptoms:

Pain: The pain of fibromyalgia has no boundaries. People describe the pain as deep muscular aching, burning, throbbing, shooting, and stabbing. Quite often, the pain and stiffness are worse in the morning. Muscle groups that are used repetitively may be particularly painful.

Fatigue: This symptom can be mild in some patients and incapacitating in others. The fatigue has been described as "brain fatigue," in which patients feel totally drained of energy. Concentration is difficult.

Sleep disorder: Most fibromyalgia patients have an associated sleep disorder called the alpha-EEG anomaly. This condition was uncovered in a sleep lab with the aid of a machine that recorded the brain waves of patients during sleep. Researchers found that FMS patients could fall asleep without much trouble, but their deep-level (or stage 4) sleep was constantly interrupted by bursts of awake-like brain activity. If you wake up feeling tired from what doctors refer to as unrefreshed sleep, it is reasonable for your physician to assume that you have a sleep disorder. It should be noted that most patients diagnosed with chronic fatigue syndrome have the same alpha-EEG sleep pattern and some fibromyalgia-diagnosed patients have been found to have other sleep disorders, such as sleep myoclonus or PLMS (nighttime jerking of the arms and legs), restless leg syndrome, and bruxism (teeth grinding).

Irritable bowel syndrome: Constipation, diarrhea, frequent abdominal pain, abdominal gas, and nausea are symptoms found in roughly 40 to 70 percent of fibromyalgia patients.

Chronic headaches: Recurrent migraine or tension-type headaches are typical in about 50 percent of fibromyalgia patients.

Temporomandibular joint dysfunction syndrome: This syndrome, sometimes referred to as TMJD, causes tremendous face and head pain. A 1997 report indicates that as many as 90 percent of fibromyalgia patients may have jaw and facial tenderness that could produce, at least intermittently, symptoms of TMJD. Most of the problems associated with this condition are thought to be related to the muscles and ligaments surrounding the joint and not necessarily the joint itself.

Multiple chemical sensitivity syndrome: Sensitivities to odors, noise, bright lights, medications, and various foods are common in roughly 50 percent of FMS patients.

Other common symptoms: Painful menstrual periods (dysmenorrhea), chest pain, morning stiffness, cognitive or memory impairment, numbness and tingling sensations, muscle twitching, irritable bladder, the feeling of swollen extremities, skin sensitivities, dry eyes and mouth, frequent changes in eye prescription, dizziness, and impaired coordination can occur.

Multiple Sclerosis

Multiple sclerosis (MS) is a disease in which the immune system targets nerve tissues of the central nervous system. Progress of the disease is marked by decreased nerve function with initial inflammation of the myelin sheath. Myelin is a layer that forms around nerves. Its purpose is to speed the transmission of impulses along nerve cells. Inflammation slows or blocks the transmission of nerve impulses in that area, leading to the symptoms of MS.

Symptoms and severity of symptoms vary widely because the location and extent of each attack varies. MS may progress into episodes of crisis that last days, weeks, or months and alternate with episodes of remission. Most commonly, damage to the central nervous system occurs intermittently, allowing a person to lead a fairly normal life. At the other extreme, the symptoms may become constant, resulting in a progressive disease with possible blindness, paralysis, and premature death.

Rheumatoid Arthritis

In people with rheumatoid arthritis, the immune system predominantly targets the lining (synovium) that covers various joints. Inflammation of the synovium usually occurs equally on both sides of the body and causes pain, swelling, and stiffness of the joints. These features distinguish rheumatoid arthritis from osteoarthritis, the more common, degenerative, "wear-and-tear" arthritis.

Rheumatoid arthritis is a systemic disease, capable of attacking other parts of the body besides the joints. Because of this systemic involvement, people with rheumatoid arthritis may experience fatigue even though there are no specific joint complaints. The nervous system may also be affected. In some cases, compression of peripheral nerves results in sensory changes or loss or in motor function diminishment, resulting in a "dropped" hand or foot. In cases where there is involvement of the cervical vertebrae, spinal cord compression can occur.

Various lesions of the eye may occur, including some that are painful. Some patients may develop "dry eyes."

Rheumatoid nodules and other skin problems may develop in certain people with the disease. The nodules develop in approximately 25 percent of patients, usually those with the most rapidly progressive form of the disease. Those with nodules are likely to develop them in areas of the body where pressure is applied, like the sacrum (the part of the back connected to the pelvis) and elbows. The patient's skin can also become fragile (easily torn) and bruise easily.

Some people with rheumatoid arthritis may develop obstructive-type lung disease. Other patients may develop pericarditis (inflammation of the membrane surrounding the heart) as a result. Less commonly, other disorders of the cardiopulmonary system can occur.

Involvement of major body organs is also possible. Enlargement of the spleen, anemia, and abnormal enlargement of the lymph nodes may result from the disease. These pathological changes in conjunction with fever, fatigue, anorexia, and weight loss are known as Felty's syndrome.

Systemic Lupus Erythematosus

Patients with systemic lupus erythematosus most commonly experience profound fatigue, rashes, and joint pains. In severe cases, the immune system may attack and damage organs such as the kidney, brain, or lung. Infections are found in an extremely high percentage of people who have lupus. People with lupus (or another autoimmune disease) often have more than one type: bacterial, viral, and/or from various types of parasitic bacteria called mycoplasma. In some cases, these infections are opportunistic. In other words, they occur because the immune system has been wiped out by lupus and can't fight off these infections. For many individuals, symptoms and damage from the disease can be controlled with anti-inflammatory medications. However, if a patient is not closely monitored, the side effects from the medications can be quite serious.

Inflammatory Conditions

A collection of immune system cells and molecules at a target site is broadly referred to as inflammation. Inflammatory conditions are common among women with endometriosis, including the following reported problems.

Asthma

Asthma is a disease of the lungs that obstructs the airways. During an asthma attack, muscle spasms constrict the bronchial tubes in the lungs, impeding the ability to expel air. These spasms are a result of chronic inflammation and hypersensitivity of the bronchial airways to particular triggers. Triggers cause airways to swell and become plugged with mucus, increasing inflammation. Triggers may include:

- allergens (like pollen or house dust);
- irritants (like tobacco smoke or air pollution);
- exercise; and
- respiratory infections.

Asthma is often accompanied by wheezing, shortness of breath, tightness in the chest, and coughing, particularly at night or in the early morning. With asthma, some inflammation is always present, but symptoms may disappear between attacks.

Interstitial Cystitis

Interstitial cystitis (IC), a chronic inflammation of the bladder wall not caused by bacteria, results in recurring discomfort or pain in the bladder and the surrounding pelvic region. The symptoms of IC vary from case to case and even in the same individual. People may experience mild discomfort, pressure, tenderness, or intense pain in the bladder and surrounding pelvic area. Symptoms may include an urgent need to urinate (urgency), frequent need to urinate (frequency), or a combination of these symptoms. Pain may change in intensity as the bladder fills with urine or as it empties. Women's symptoms often get worse during menstruation. Also, people with IC often experience pain during sexual intercourse. Pinpoint bleeding caused by recurrent irritation may appear on the bladder wall, contributing to scarring.

Some people with IC find that their bladders cannot hold much urine, which increases the frequency of urination. People with severe cases of IC may urinate as many as sixty times a day. Of the more than 700,000 Americans estimated to have IC, 90 percent are women.

In IC, the protective layer is denuded, allowing substances such as potassium to filter across the usually impermeable bladder wall. The result is pain from nerve-ending excitation and, ultimately, mast cell migration and degranulation. This leads to a vicious cycle of chronic pain. People with endometriosis, vulvar vestibulitis, irritable bowel syndrome (IBS), and IC have similar symptoms. These patients typically complain of cyclic pain associated with hormone fluctuation; symptoms flaring around the time of menstruation or after intercourse; pain throughout the lower abdomen, genital area, and thighs; and, very often, urinary symptoms. A new method of diagnosing IC that is becoming increasingly popular is the potassium sensitivity challenge (PSC). One study demonstrated that 90 percent of people with symptoms of IC have a positive PSC result. Another study showed that as many as 89 percent of patients with CPP (chronic pelvic pain) presumed to be from endometriosis had a positive PSC, indicating that their bladder pain was possibly from IC.

Estrogen deficiencies may also lead to urinary tract symptoms. The lower urinary tract depends on estrogen. When supplies are depleted— common in women with endometriosis because one treatment for endo is reducing estrogen levels—the urethral tissues atrophy (shrink), followed by incontinence.

Vaginitis

Vaginitis is an inflammatory condition in the vagina that is primarily the result of infection (i.e., from Candida albicans, Trichomonas vaginalis, Gardnerella vaginalis, or Chlamydia trachomatis) or exposure to an irritant (chemical or allergic). The symptoms of vaginitis generally include an abnormal vaginal discharge and itching or burning.

One of the most common types of vaginitis is a yeast infection, usually caused by the yeast Candida albicans. The vagina normally is populated by a variety of microorganisms that help to prevent infection. The beneficial microorganisms create a chemical environment that inhibits the harmful microorganisms. When a woman takes antibiotics to treat any infection, whether for vaginitis or something else, the antibiotics kill both the bad and the good microorganisms. The vagina can normally exist comfortably with small amounts of yeast, but the killing of good microorganisms by antibiotics allows yeast to grow significantly, creating a yeast infection. Other factors that can disrupt the balance of microorganisms in the vagina are a high-sugar diet, birth control pills, and certain hormonal changes, including those caused by pregnancy.

Environmental Toxins and Endometriosis: Food for Thought

Dioxins formed during the manufacture and incineration of such chlorine-based substances as vinyl (polyvinyl chloride, or PVC) are released into the air and travel via air currents, contaminating fields and crops as they land. When cattle and other livestock eat the crops, dioxin enters their tissues, thus becoming part of the food chain. When consumed by people, dioxin becomes a player in human biochemistry. The implications of this biochemical invasion may have profound consequences on overall human reproductive health and on endometriosis in particular.

In the early 1990s, the Endometriosis Association reported that 79 percent of a group of monkeys developed endometriosis after exposure to dioxin in their food during a research study begun more than ten years earlier. The severity of endometriosis found in the monkeys was directly related to the amount of TCDD (2,3,7,8-tetrachlorodibenzo-p-dioxin, the most toxic dioxin) to which they had been exposed. Monkeys that were fed dioxin in amounts as small as five parts per trillion developed endometriosis. In addition, the dioxin-exposed monkeys showed immune abnormalities similar to those observed in women with endometriosis.

As explained in *The Endometriosis Sourcebook* (1995) and other sources, scientists have come to the realization that certain chemical compounds, such as dioxin, have profound immunological and reproductive effects at exposures far below the level known to cause cancer. These chemicals are known as endocrine disruptors and can mimic hormones and interfere with many physiological processes. Scientists already know that these synthetic chemicals persist in the body for years. PCBs (polychlorinated biphenyls) are a group of dioxin-like chemicals that were widely used in industry until they were banned in the 1970s. Some PCBs persist in the environment for more than one hundred years. According to Endometriosis Association research, certain PCBs appear to be linked with TCDD in endometriosis in the monkeys.

According to animal studies and observation of wildlife, impaired fertility is another result of exposure to endocrine disruptors. Infertility affects approximately 40 percent of women with endometriosis. (See Chapter Nine for in-depth discussion of fertility issues.) The Endometriosis Association's research registry provides data showing that endometriosis is starting at a younger age and is more severe than in the past. The question for future research: could this be the result of a more burdensome level of dioxins and other endocrine disruptors?

Because recent research into endometriosis is establishing links to the importance of the immune system in the development and management of endometriosis, Chapter Seven explores some natural immune-enhancing strategies. Of course, sound nutrition may be the body's best defense of all. Learn more in Chapter Eight.

Don't Despair!

Of course, no one will experience all of the illnesses and symptoms described here. I included them in the book because it's important to make links between your certain symptoms and the problems they might point to. A woman usually has symptoms of a combination of illnesses and, knowing this, she and her doctor can create a health program that takes into consideration all of the conditions that affect the quality of her life.

A PERSONAL STORY

Maria

"I always knew I had something wrong," Maria starts, classic words of women who have conditions like endometriosis. Maria's "something wrong" was to suffer through a lot of pain in silence.

Her periods were "bad—painful with a heavy flow." Maria recalls that in those first years of menstruation, she had to bring a change of clothes to school in case she soiled the clothes she wore to school that morning. They were difficult years. "I would go the whole month," she recalls, "having only two or three days each month where I was pain-free."

Two or three days out of each month is no way to live life to its fullest. But Maria simply toughed it out until she had difficulty getting pregnant.

When Maria first got married, she and her husband wanted to wait to have a child and she took birth control pills. The pain and other symptoms (of endometriosis, but she didn't have a diagnosis yet) subsided. When they were ready to start a family, she went off the pill and had her first child, with no problems getting pregnant. When they tried for a second child, Maria couldn't get pregnant. After eight months of trying, she went to a fertility specialist, the first real step toward diagnosis for many women with endometriosis (and other conditions) to find out what had been plaguing them all these years.

The visit with the fertility specialist had its good and bad moments. She heard about endometriosis for the first time. Her fertility doctor diagnosed her and did laparoscopic surgery. It was a six-hour operation; her ovaries were in very bad condition. He told her she was a "stage 4" but didn't give her any details. He did the best surgery job he could, he said.

"He never told me that the endometriosis was wrapped around my bowels," Maria recalls. Even after the surgery, she got progressively worse. Her doctor put her on another round of fertility drugs, but they did not do any good. A whole month of Maria's life was just a blur.

A friend encouraged Maria to contact Dr. Lyons, but Maria had absolutely no intention of traveling from her home in New Jersey to Atlanta. She lived near New York City, after all—who couldn't find the best doctors in the New York metropolitan area? And she never had any intention of having laparoscopic surgery again.

"But my friend insisted I at least call, so I did," she says. "He was so reassuring, there is this real comfort zone when you talk with him. He first told me to forget about having a baby for the time being, that from my descriptions and symptoms and history he thought my endometriosis was way worse than I imagined and that I first needed to concentrate on taking care of myself."

"My family all thought I was crazy to go to Atlanta, but after I hung up, I just had this feeling."

And so off she went to Atlanta. Maria had a bowel resection using laser surgery and she had excisional surgery for all the endometriosis removing all the visible disease. She flew home just two days after the surgery, and then proceeded to get pregnant and have triplets!

After the triplets were born, Maria again had pain once her periods started coming back. Dr. Lyons had warned her that this might happen and she called him to talk it over.

Maria decided to return to Atlanta for a hysterectomy. Three years later, she is feeling great. She has since come to love the city of Atlanta, and she has also referred a couple of friends to the center.

Maria definitely has advice for women who are suffering with endometriosis or, if they are not yet diagnosed, with endo-like symptoms.

"You absolutely need to find someone with whom you are comfortable and who takes you seriously. Learn what you can—I spent a lot of time online on Websites. Find a good surgeon. This is a debilitating disease. Above all, do whatever it takes to get this level of care for yourself."

Even if it means a couple of trips from New Jersey to Atlanta!

CHAPTER SEVEN ∽

Natural Approaches
Relieving Pain, Treating Symptoms

Because endometriosis is a chronic, multi-symptom challenge to well-being, awareness of any and every possible approach to managing symptoms is an important key to improved health and quality of life. Many women with endometriosis have discovered the power of alternative and natural therapies to reduce symptoms, enhance the immune system, diminish physical pain, and improve emotional balance.

This chapter offers an overview of complementary therapies that have established track records for relieving a variety of symptoms that women with endometriosis may confront. Natural healing therapies offer many options for improved health, but—just like conventional therapies—finding the right combination for you may require homework, time, and experimentation.

Keep in mind that a remedy or approach that worked wonders for your neighbor might not noticeably improve your symptoms. But don't give up. The odds are in your favor that another approach or combination of approaches will provide some measure of relief.

And even though natural remedies are considered safe and typically do not carry the potential side effects of synthetic drugs, always keep your doctor and the rest of your health care team apprised of any natural remedies you are taking (see more about pulling together your health care team in Chapter 11). Most physicians are experienced with patients choosing to explore holistic options. Some patients work with a holistic practitioner.

There is a reasonable chance that some natural therapies can cross-react with traditional medical therapies, and it may be of real importance to anticipate and control these reactions. So be wise and talk about all of these areas with your doctor so that optimal results can be obtained with the least amount of risk or side effects. The complexity of endometriosis and the level of pain often experienced requires you to look at all angles!

So where do you start? Let's look at some of the advantages of incorporating natural approaches into treating endometriosis.

What's in a Name?

First, here's a definition of two oft-repeated words regarding herbs, energy therapies, and other natural approaches: alternative and complementary. Complementary and alternative therapies can be understood as therapeutic practices that are not currently integrated into conventional Western medical practice. Therapies are termed complementary when used in addition to conventional treatment and alternative when used instead of conventional treatment. A good example would be acupuncture. For years, acupuncture would have been considered an alternative treatment because it often was used in place of traditional therapies. Today, acupuncture is often used along with other, more traditional modes of treatment and therefore would be considered complementary. So it's largely how you and your team choose to use natural approaches that defines them.

Why Try Natural Options?

Natural or holistic approaches to healing are usually non-invasive and typically free of unpleasant side effects. Medicines in natural therapies are derived from natural substances, usually plants or minerals. Many healing therapies are quite relaxing, which may interrupt the cycle of pain, tension, and depression that often accompanies life with endometriosis. Improved feelings of well-being alone are known to boost the immune system and may help your body to better resist endo. And some women find that the focused attention offered by complementary therapists is in itself extremely therapeutic. In short, attention and touch by themselves are therapeutic.

Most complementary medical therapies are holistic, exploring all facets of healing—including the physical, mental, and emotional aspects—to stimulate the body's innate ability to overcome disease. Compared to approaches that focus solely on treatment of symptoms, alternative therapies place a heavy emphasis on prevention. Broadly speaking, the goal of holistic therapies is to promote balance. Many practitioners offer advice on nutrition, lifestyle, and coping strategies to enhance the effectiveness of therapy.

Complementary therapies not usually offered by the general medical system include a wide range of options, such as herbal medicine, homeopathy, acupuncture, chiropractic, and naturopathy. Historically, mainstream doctors have not typically worked closely with complementary therapists, although an important sign of the growing acceptance of natural approaches is that some medical schools have begun offering courses on alternative medicine. Western physicians tend to rely heavily on research results in their practices, and although many natural therapies lack a large body of research (research is expensive), chiropractic, naturopathy, and traditional Chinese medicine (TCM) are reasonably well researched. Research on herbs and vitamins does continue to accumulate as interest (and therefore funding for research) increases in the West. Anecdotal evidence about the effectiveness of natural therapies is widespread.

An Exciting New Study

In late 2001, the Oregon College of Oriental Medicine (OCOM) was awarded a $250,000 grant by the National Center for Complementary and Alternative Medicine. The grant, according the news release on the OCOM web site, is the first of its kind awarded to a school of Oriental medicine, and will fund a two-year research project comparing the effectiveness of TCM versus hormone therapy in relieving chronic pain related to endometriosis.

In the study, 66 women with endometriosis diagnosed through laparoscopy will be randomly assigned to one of two groups. The first group will receive conventional hormone therapy; the other group will receive TCM in the form of acupuncture and an herbal formula. Check the OCOM web site (www.ocom.edu) for the latest news on this exciting study, which is intended to be used to design a large-scale research trial. Cost will be an issue in this research, however, so don't expect too much. Also, the current methods of evaluating pain and the surrounding responses are very subjective and can be difficult to interpret.

Working With a Complementary Therapist

Your active participation in alternative approaches is often a central part of the natural healing process. Be sure to investigate the world of holistic therapies; some great books are listed in the resource section. The Internet offers instant access to information and ideas of interest, as well as to practitioners, but like anything else on the Internet, you need to be aware of the credibility of the source. Your local endometriosis support group may be the perfect place to meet other women and learn about their experiences with complementary therapies.

Here are some suggestions for working with a natural care provider:

- Seek a licensed therapist. If there are no national certification boards in your area, look for a therapist who is a member of a local association and committed to the profession. There are certainly many natural approaches you can do yourself, but with a condition like endometriosis, it would be best to work with a trained therapist.

• For the best, most comprehensive care and for safety and health reasons, discuss all your complementary treatments and therapies with your doctor. Likewise, discuss all medications you may be taking with your complementary therapist. It isn't beneficial to you to not mention something—if you are taking an herbal treatment, by all means tell your medical doctor! You are the ultimate control factor in your health care, so you should be sure to bring up anything you are taking (for endometriosis or anything else). If your doctor demeans your holistic efforts, you might want to find a different doctor who is more sympathetic to natural approaches. And if your doctor is concerned about an herb or homeopathic treatment, be sure to contact your naturopath to discuss this concern.

When you first consult with a complementary therapist, bring a list of questions, including the following.

• How does the therapy work?
• Have you used this therapy specifically for treating endometriosis?
• What evidence does this therapy have for its claims of success?
• What results can I anticipate?
• How long is the therapy effective?
• What will it cost and is it covered by medical insurance?
• Will I need to suspend other forms of treatment and medications?

As with your conventional medical doctor, your comfort with the answers you receive and your degree of confidence in the practitioner are good indicators for whether or not to begin a particular treatment. Keep in mind that, unlike Western approaches, natural therapies are more subtle in effect and typically take some time before benefits are apparent. Once treatment begins, you should notice results within a time span ranging from a few weeks or to six months. Your practitioner will monitor your responses and make adjustments and recommendations as necessary.

The following section offers introductory overviews of various alternative approaches, including the benefits you might expect for specific endometriosis symptoms. There is a lot more information to know about each approach, so use this list as a basic guide and then investigate further the ones that interest you. Keep in mind that combining approaches in your healing process—for instance, practicing yoga along with taking herbs—may yield multiple benefits for symptom relief and overall improved health. Work with your practitioner to design a program that addresses your individual issues.

Acupuncture Basics

Acupuncture has a history that reaches back for thousands of years. Before communication was reopened with China thirty years ago, acupuncture was extremely rare in the Western world. Today, acupuncture is a widely accepted and widely practiced medical therapy. Its use extends into mainstream medicine in the United States and throughout the world.

The TCM health system that includes acupuncture—as well as herbs, acupressure, exercise, and diet—is based in part on the concept of a universal life energy known as qi (also known as chi, ki, and prana). A person's health is said to be influenced by the flow of qi; balanced circulation of qi is understood to be essential for good health.

Qi travels throughout the body along pathways, known as meridians, located just below the surface of the skin. Energy constantly flows up and down these pathways. When meridians become blocked, deficient, or excessive, illness is the expected result. Acupuncture's goal is to restore qi circulation and bring the body back to good health.

Acupuncturists use observation, listening, questioning, and pulse taking to arrive at a diagnosis. Treatment options are discussed, followed perhaps by advice on lifestyle and diet. In some cases, Chinese herbal medicine may be recommended.

To influence the circulation of qi by stimulating or suppressing its flow, practitioners insert extremely fine, sterile, disposable needles into specific points along the meridians; there is typically no discomfort associated with insertion of these needles. There are about 365 "acupoints"—areas where the meridians pass near the surface of the skin and are easily accessible—where qi is concentrated and can enter or leave the body. The needles are typically left in place for between twenty and forty-five minutes.

Other methods of influencing acupoints might be used, including moxibusiton, which is the application of heat to acupuncture points, sometimes incorporating herbs, and cupping, a method of stimulating acupuncture points by applying suction through a special cup in which a partial vacuum has been created.

Studies have shown that acupuncture brings various degrees of relief to women suffering from pain, menstrual cramping, nausea, headache, backache, fluid retention, or post-op pain. Acupuncture releases endorphins, chemicals produced by the body that are natural painkillers and that generate a feeling of well-being. Acupuncture has also been used successfully in infertility treatment.

Biofeedback Therapy

Biofeedback therapy is an approach to relieving pain caused by muscular tension and poor circulation caused by narrowing of the blood vessel diameter. Constriction of the skeletal muscles and the smooth muscle of the blood vessel wall usually occur on an unconscious level. This constriction can worsen problems such as fibroids, endometriosis, migraine headaches, and high blood pressure.

Using biofeedback therapy, people learn to recognize when they are tensing their muscles. Wolpian relaxation techniques, which can be learned with the help of biofeedback mechanisms, aid you in abating this tension and thereby improve the underlying pain response. Once this response is understood, endometriosis sufferers can learn to relax their muscles to help relieve pain. For relief of cramps, women can learn biofeedback therapy through a series of training sessions with a trained professional, who can teach women how to consciously change their vaginal temperature. Even a slight rise in the temperature indicates better blood flow and muscle relaxation in the pelvic area, with a concomitant relief of menstrual pain.

Menstrual pain relief and stress reduction can be expected from biofeedback therapy.

Chinese Herbs

Using the diagnostic techniques listed for acupuncture, an herbalist arrives at a prescription to benefit individual symptoms. In TCM, herbs are generally taken as a formula that includes a variety of herbs, each with a different role, to treat an individual's pattern of disharmony. Herbs are most often taken in the form of tea, but capsules, powders, ointments, or lotions may also be prescribed.

According to TCM theories, endometriosis is best described by the traditional Chinese category of blood stasis syndrome with formation of abdominal lumps. The underlying causes of the blood stasis (slowing of blood flow), in turn, are mainly the syndromes of qi stagnation and coldness (impaired metabolism and circulation). Therefore, in TCM, endometriosis is usually treated by herbs that vitalize blood circulation as the primary therapy.

Pelvic pain relief, including relief of pain during intercourse, has been reported by women using Chinese herb formulas. More regular menstrual cycles and improved post-operative healing have also been reported.

Chiropractic

Chiropractic, the most widely practiced complementary health treatment in the West, focuses on manipulating and adjusting the spine and joints in other parts of the body. Chiropractic theory centers on the central role of the spine, which links the brain (regulator of the central nervous system) to the body. The autonomic nervous system within the spine regulates what we think of as automatic internal body functions like digestion and heart rate. Spinal damage or distortion can interfere with nerves, disrupting the function of internal organs, glands, and the circulatory system. Chiropractors believe that when the skeletal structure is functioning correctly, the body can marshal innate healing forces throughout the system.

Chiropractic adjustment should result in pain relief, which may be immediate or within a day or two of treatment, as well as in improvement of bowel and bladder problems. Restoring normal mobility to the pelvis can reduce soft-tissue strain. Cervical (neck) and thoracic (torso) adjustments are thought to benefit immune function.

The use of radiographic imaging (x-ray) or ultrasonography by chiropractors for diagnosis should be considered suspect, as these tests are generally not helpful in these practitioners' hands. Hydrotherapy, electrostimulatory treatment, therapeutic ultrasound, and electromagnetic therapy are all valid treatments that have been used with some success by chiropractors.

Flower Remedies

In the early part of the twentieth century, a London doctor who was also a homeopath studied his patients and concluded that negative emotions could lead to physical illness. Convinced that flowers contained healing properties he called "vibrational energy" for the emotions, Edward Bach infused flowers in spring water, retained the water, and preserved the essences in brandy. Today, Bach flower remedies are popular around the world and used primarily for self-help during times of stress or emotional turmoil.

Bach remedies are said to transform emotions such as fear, anger, guilt, and depression into positive emotions, such as optimism and joy. Remedies are generally self-prescribed based on the seven categories developed by Dr. Bach, each associated with one or more specific botanicals. He also developed a blend of five essences he called Rescue Remedy to counteract shock or panic from acute crises.

Rescue Remedy is often recommended for women with endometriosis to address stress and tension. Gorse is said to help with feelings of hopelessness, and olive is used for mental and physical exhaustion. Sweet chestnut is suggested for women who feel they have reached their limits of endurance.

Remedies can be diluted in water or fruit juice for sipping, dropped directly from the dropper onto the tongue, or misted on the body using a spray bottle. Usual dosage is four drops of solution four times a day. Rescue Remedy can be taken every five minutes or so until acute feelings of panic or shock subside.

Managing stress is now known to be a key factor in overall health, either from chronic illness or life's stresses in general. The emotional relief that Bach flower remedies address may be one more aid in relieving the stress of dealing with endometriosis.

Herbal Medicine

Herbal (also known as botanical) medicines have been made from flowers, roots, leaves, stems, seeds, and bark throughout recorded history. Many conventional drugs, like digitalis and aspirin, are derived from botanicals, although most Western pharmaceuticals are based on synthetic versions (you can't patent things that exist naturally!). Side effects, including addiction, from herbs are uncommon, although nothing is impossible. Remedies typically combine several herbs for maximum benefit.

Various herbs said to be helpful in relieving endometriosis pain include blue cohosh, cranberry, cayenne, plantain, St. John's Wort, peppermint, valerian, dong quai, false unicorn, evening primrose oil, black cohosh, couchgrass, red raspberry, and white willow (a precursor to aspirin). Work with a trained herbalist to identify the combination and dosages appropriate for you. (CAUTION: Dong quai is not recommended for women with excessive menstrual flow. Avoid hormone-balancing herbs if you are taking birth control pills, fertility drugs, hormone replacement therapy or other hormonal treatment, or other medication unless recommended by an experienced herbal practitioner. The following list is for informational purposes. It bears repeating that you should always work with both your medical doctor and herbalist to find the best treatment for your specific issues.)

- Dong quai, an aromatic herb that grows in China, Korea, and Japan, is frequently used in TCM as a strengthening treatment for the heart, spleen, liver, and kidneys. Dong quai contains vitamins A, B12, and E. Researchers have isolated at least six derivatives that exert antispasmodic effects, helping in relieving menstrual cramps. Elements in this herb can prevent spasms, reduce blood clotting, and relax peri-pheral blood vessels. Research has shown that dong quai produces a balancing effect on estrogen activity.

- Goldenseal and shepherd's purse have been shown to be effective in regulating heavy menstrual bleeding.

- Wild yam can alleviate pain in the lower abdomen.

- Chamomile flowers and rosemary may relieve menstrual and pre-menstrual pain.

- Slippery elm and ginger root can counteract the irritating effects on the stomach that some people experience from some synthetic drugs.

- Agnus castus (Vitex/Chastetree berry) is an important herb for female hormone imbalances. The pituitary gland controls and balances the hormones in the body. Agnus castus works to restore pituitary balance by stimulating progesterone production.

- Echinacea (Echinacea purpurea) is the herb of choice for the immune system; it helps to increase white blood cell count.

- Ginseng has been shown to enhance the overall activity of the im-mune system, as well as reduce fatigue.

- For aches and pains, try peppermint tea. Peppermint tea is an effective antispasmodic and muscle relaxant. It is also healthy for the liver. Because the liver is responsible for breaking down estrogen, it has been suggested that poor liver function may be implicated in the flare of endometriosis. If treated, improved liver function can have a relieving effect on symptoms, in part by removing excess levels of estrogen. Other herbs that support liver health include dandelion, beet leaves, cascara, and uva ursi. Milk thistle (Silybum marianum) is an excellent herb for the liver, which needs to work efficiently to balance the hormones. A number of studies have shown that milk thistle can result in an increase in new liver cells to replace damaged cells.

Homeopathy

Homeopathic medicine follows the "principle of similars." According to this principle, when large doses of a substance cause symptoms, the same substance can heal when given in tiny, specially prepared doses. It is estimated that about 500 million people worldwide use homeopathic remedies. There are more than two thousand homeopathic preparations, based on plant, animal, and mineral compounds. Remedies in the United States are made under U.S. Food and Drug Administration (FDA) regulation, and manufacturers adhere to strict standards.

According to Michael Carlston, MD, a homeopath and assistant clinical professor at the University of California at San Francisco School of Medicine, homeopathic medicines can be very helpful in the early and middle stages of endometriosis. However, because of heavy scarring during advanced stages of the disease, remedies may be less effective for severe endometriosis. In truth, because of the elusive origin of endo and the source of pain being difficult to ascertain, homeopathic remedies that exceed the normal rate of placebo effect are rare indeed.

Homeopathic remedies are said to be able to boost immune health, balance hormones, and reduce pain and inflammation. (NOTE: Endometriosis is not amenable to self-care; professional homeopathic care is recommended.)

Naturopathy

Naturopathic treatment takes an integrative approach, focusing on diet, lifestyle, a positive outlook, and preventive measures to treat underlying causes of illness and emphasize achieving good health. Naturopathic physicians are trained as primary care physicians and use both conventional and alternative methods of diagnosis. Treatment aims to eliminate toxins from the body (detoxification) and rebuild the immune system so that good health becomes dominant. Detoxification of the body is encouraged with diet changes, fasts, fruit juices, and mineral water. The primary goal is to promote the healing process; treatments may include massage, hydrotherapy, use of supplements, chiropractic, homeopathy, TCM, and lifestyle changes and are tailored to individual needs based on these cleansing and strengthening principles.

Two endometriosis-related benefits that could result from the naturopathic approach are balancing hormones and resolving systemic Candida albicans infections through dietary changes and supplementation.

The therapeutic goal of naturopathic approaches is to enhance the body's innate ability to maintain good health. The naturopathic approach has been endorsed by current medical research. Working with one physician who oversees a range of complementary treatments may simplify the healing process.

Rolfing

Rolfing is a form of deep tissue body work that improves body posture, energy levels, mobility, and circulation. The connective tissue, or myofascial system, that supports the soft tissues of the body, including organs, determines the spacing and positioning of bones and the direction of muscle pulls and movement and gives the body its shape. Deep-tissue treatments focus on stretching and lengthening the fascia to restore pliability and efficiency of movement and increase mobility. Releasing fascial tension can markedly improve energy levels. Some women with endometriosis have claimed that Rolfing produced profound relief from the pain caused by adhesions. Again, there is no substantiation of this in clinical research, but anecdotal information is available.

Shiatsu

Shiatsu, considered a catalyst in the healing process, is based on the principles of TCM and aims to regulate the flow of energy along the meridian pathways through pressure and massage. Massage aims to release toxins and deep tensions from the muscles and stimulate the hormone system, enhancing a sense of well-being and pain relief, as well as reducing feelings of stress and depression.

Shiatsu practitioners in the West say that this therapy can regulate the hormonal system, improve blood and lymph circulation, improve the body's ability to eliminate toxins, release muscle tension, and promote deep relaxation. Shiatsu practitioners consider endometriosis to be a blood stagnation condition and may focus on stimulating the liver and spleen meridians in the legs to enhance circulation. Exercises to practice at home may be recommended.

Yoga

Yoga practice centers around specific postures, breathing techniques, and relaxation exercises. Yoga may improve flexibility, suppleness, and blood circulation and oxygenation in muscles, which may be severely impeded by pain and cramping. Yoga postures not only develop flexibility in the spine and back, reducing pain, they also balance the hormone system and may promote health in the immune system. The slow, deliberate movements encouraged in yoga practice are less likely to trigger pain in adhesions. Certain postures may reduce cyclical issues like premenstrual tension, lower back pain, and menstrual pain. And there are emotional benefits as well. Modified breathing patterns play a role in creating mental and emotional harmony. The deep breathing and quiet movements reduce anxiety and stress levels and produce feelings of peace, related to the release of the body's "feel-good" chemicals, endorphins. Yoga has been helpful in pain reduction. Estrogen is stored in fat, so a regular exercise program is essential for any woman needing to balance hormone levels. Yoga is an excellent addition to the exercise regimen of any woman with endometriosis.

Yoga can be particularly helpful for people with rheumatoid arthritis. Regular yoga practice can tone muscles and keep stiffness at bay. The American Yoga Association and the Arthritis Foundation have co-produced a guide called Remain Active with RA that outlines a program to improve range of motion, muscle strength, and endurance. Contact the Arthritis Foundation at (800) 283-7800 for more information.

Putting it all Together: Relief for a Few Common Symptoms

As is true of most of the therapies just described, strengthening the overall immune system in general—and sometimes specific organic systems—is the backbone of natural approaches to health. A few natural self-help strategies, targeted at specific common symptoms, are described in the following sections. I hope that these strategies give you some ideas for simple changes that could make a big difference in your day-to-day life. If natural approaches appeal to you and as you expand your investigation of natural approaches, chances are you'll discover a world that also offers relief for many other endometriosis symptoms.

Keep in mind that good health requires good nutrition—especially for chronic conditions—and nutrition really is the foundation of a natural approach to health. (See Chapter Eight.) So eat well to feed your body, mind, and spirit and then build on that foundation with natural tactics for relief from specific symptoms of endo-metriosis. You can dabble if you want, but it is highly recommended that you consult with a licensed nutritionist, naturopath, or other qualified health care professional to help you identify the most appropriate supplemental or nutritional plan for the best quality of life possible.

Allergy Relief

Many people with allergies have found relief through using bee pollen, which reduces the production of the histamine that can cause allergic responses. Eating bee pollen can strengthen the respiratory system and provides protein that can help the body build a natural defense shield against allergic responses. Also, bee pollen is rapidly absorbed into the bloodstream to stimulate immune responses. It has also proved beneficial for nausea and sleep disorders.

The Chinese herb called immature bitter orange contains a powerful antioxidant called nobelitin that helps this herb combat allergies and other inflammatory conditions.

The homeopathic remedy Euphrasia is recommended in the early stages of allergic symptoms and is said to especially good for watery, itchy eyes.

Although it sounds like some toxic chemical that you would find near an old nuclear power plant, methylsulfonylmethane (MSM) is an easily absorbable form of organic sulfur found in botanicals, meat, eggs, poultry, and dairy foods. From it, the body manufactures important enzymes, antibodies, amino acids, antioxidants, and connective tissue. The processing that most of our foods go through can destroy much of the sulfur content of foods, and deficiencies can lead to many health problems.

Supplementation with MSM has shown to be particularly effective in reducing or even eliminating allergy symptoms. (It has reduced asthma symptoms, too, and also possesses anti-inflammatory characteristics.) Two 1000 mg tablets daily with food is the recommended amount.

Zapping Yeast Infections

Yeast infection, usually caused by Candida albicans, is one of the most common types of vaginitis. Factors that can disrupt the ecological balance in the vagina, allowing Candida to flourish, are a high-sugar diet, extended antibiotic use, allergies, birth control pills, and certain hormonal changes, including those caused by pregnancy. As yeasts multiply beyond normal limits, they release toxins that affect many metabolic processes and further tax the immune system. The endocrine, digestive, and nervous systems are considered especially susceptible to yeast-related overloads. Health problems related to Candida overload can best be addressed by a special diet and antifungal medication, according to Dr. William Crook in his book *The Yeast Connection*. Dr. Crook offers a wide spectrum of sugar-free, yeast-free strategies and recipes for dealing with Candida. Although the best long-term strategies for overcoming yeast infections may involve changes in diet and perhaps your environment, there are some natural strategies for zapping vaginitis caused by Candida albicanis.

Homeopathic medicines can strengthen a woman's own defenses, which help her body fight off the infection, without disturbing internal flora balance like antibiotics do. Some of the common remedies for vaginitis include the following:

Borax: for a burning vaginal discharge which is the color of egg whites; borax tends to be useful for vaginitis that occurs midway between menstrual periods.

Pulsatilla: for white, yellow, or greenish bland vaginal discharge with vaginal soreness.

Kreosotum: for itching with burning pains; a yellow, putrid vaginal discharge that irritates the vaginal lips and surrounding skin; the discharge may stain bed sheets and is worse in the morning and upon standing.

Hydrastis: for profuse stringy yellow vaginal discharge with great itching, worse after menstruation.

Sepia: for white, milky, offensive, itchy, and burning discharge that tends to be more profuse in the morning and while walking, accompanied by general fatigue, constipation, irritability, depression, and sensations of uncomfortable pressure and heaviness in the vaginal area.

Graphites: for premenstrual yeast infection, with thin, white, acrid discharge accompanied by a backache; increased discharge in the morning and while walking.

Calcarea carb: for thick yellow or milky discharge that tends to cause intense itching, worse before menses; a headache and spasmodic cramps may be concurrent.

These remedies are effective not only for yeast infections, but also for other types of vaginal infection. Seek professional homeopathic care for chronic or recurrent vaginitis.

Among the herbal remedies, aloe vera is helpful for healing infections. Apply the gel to affected skin to relieve itching or use aloe vera juice as a douche. Effective douches can be made by brewing a strong tea from one of the following herbs: calendula, goldenseal, pau d'arco, or marshmallow root. Douche twice daily for a week. Drinking pau d'arco tea three times a day may also resolve Candida infections.

Supplemental selenium (200 mcg daily) has proven helpful in helping the body withstand exposure to some environmental toxins, which may be linked to Candida proliferation.

Improving Sleep Quality
Disrupted sleep is a common complaint among women with endometriosis and Candida. Poor sleep contributes to poor health. Deep-level (stage 4) sleep is crucial for many body functions, such as tissue repair, antibody production, and perhaps even the regulation of various neurotransmitters, hormones, and immune system chemicals.

Supplements that effectively treat insomnia include those containing melatonin (a hormone produced by the pineal gland, responsible in part for the body's "internal clock") and serotonin (a chemical messenger that plays a role in bringing on sleep).

5-HTP enhances the activity of serotonin. Low levels of this hormone are associated with depression, anxiety, and sleep disorders. Since serotonin is the precursor to melatonin, the hormone that regulates sleeping and waking cycles, a boost in serotonin can improve the quality of sleep.

Tea made from hop flowers may decrease pain, stress, and anxiety and induce sleep. Valerian root tea is another herbal remedy for improving sleep. Research has shown that valerian helps improve sleep quality without the "hangover" effect of some sleep medications. Suggested nutritional supplements to improve sleep quality include magnesium, calcium, and vitamin B6.

Try visualization techniques for triggering sleep, even if you wake up at 3 am and can't get back to sleep. Concentrate on relaxing and visualize a place you find calming—the beach where waves gently lap the shore, a babbling stream in the shade of the woods. Maybe for you, the most relaxing place is in the bulkhead seat of a 757. Whatever it is, envision it and go there in your mind. Remember to breathe steadily, deeply, and rhythmically. Any number of books deal with insomnia and have helpful tips on visualization and other techniques for relaxing to fall sleep or to get back to sleep if you are awakened.

Incorporate Natural Approaches

Don't be afraid to incorporate natural approaches to healing into your endometriosis care plan. Be sure to talk with your doctor and inform your entire medical team about any approach you decide on and any treatment you are using. You need to feel comfortable taking control of your own care while at the same time taking into consideration all the experts on your team—that's what they're there for!

CHAPTER EIGHT ∾

Nutrition and Exercise

You don't have to become so fanatical about nutrition that you get a chemistry set and analyze the chemical makeup of every item of food before you put it in your mouth. But you at least will want to become well-versed in the principles of good nutrition. Later in this chapter I'll discuss some specific aspects of nutrition that a woman with endometriosis would want consider.

The Basics of Good Nutrition

Once you begin to be more conscious of nutrition and the effects that certain foods have on your body, eating well becomes a bit of an addiction in itself. Once you change your eating habits, your body's metabolism starts to change, and you won't even be tempted by foods that don't fit into your good eating habits. This is especially helpful if you are looking to lose weight, the importance of which we will discuss later in this chapter.

Though you probably won't run out and get a degree in dietary science, every adult should know some basics about the food we eat, how our bodies use that food, and what our bodies need to function optimally. And when you are faced with a health concern like endometriosis, you will want to learn a little more than the average adult about nutrition. As you know, many diseases and disorders—diabetes is perhaps the most commonly known one—are greatly affected by your eating habits and food choices.

In the United States, the American Dietetic Association (and in Canada, the ADA's counterpart, the Canadian Dietetic Association) is a major source of dietary information and guidelines. Although there are forty nutrients that food provides us, they are divided into the following six groups:

Carbohydrates: Your body gets its energy from carbohydrates. Simple carbohydrates, in the form of sugars, provide immediate energy. Complex carbohydrates come into the body in the form of starch and are processed by the digestive system into useable energy by the body. Fiber is also a carbohydrate, but is used by the body only to help the digestive process and is not a nutrient absorbed by the body.

Fats: With the nonstop discussion of cholesterol, almost everyone has heard of saturated and unsaturated fats. First, cholesterol is required by your body to perform many functions important to hormones and nutrient use. However, the human body makes all the cholesterol it needs; any extra cholesterol in the body is converted to fat. Saturated fats also contain dietary cholesterol. Excess cholesterol in the bloodstream collects around the walls of the arteries and causes arterio-sclerosis, leading to heart attack or stroke. Apart from decreasing your intake of saturated fats (from animal sources and hydrogenated oils in processed foods), another wise move is to make sure that the fats you do consume are predominantly health-promoting unsaturated fats such as olive oil (monounsaturated) and flax or cold-water fish oils (omega-3 polyunsaturated). Fats are the most concentrated source of calories (twice as many calories per gram as either carbohydrates or proteins) and should be consumed sparingly. While being conscious of the calories, it is both possible and desirable to consume small amounts of healthy fats, even if you are adhering to a dietary regimen that promotes weight loss.

Proteins: Amino acids build and repair body tissue and are critical to good health. Proteins supply amino acids to our bodies. Proteins also supply an energy boost if the body doesn't have other energy supplies to draw on.

Vitamins: Each vitamin has a different critical function in the body. They are responsible for the chemical reactions that take place to make our bodies work. Taking multi-vitamins is good thing if you feel your diet is lacking; however, the best way to bring vitamins into our bodies is via the foods we eat.

Minerals: Minerals, like vitamins, have several key roles in the proper functioning of the human body. Perhaps the most famous of the minerals is calcium, well-known for its role in bone development and health. Many other minerals are required only in trace amounts, but are still critical to human health. Deficiencies in certain trace minerals have been linked with pre-menstrual syndrome (also referred to as pre-menstrual dysphoric disorder, PMDD).

Water: Water is also essential to nutrition. Although some have questioned the old rule of thumb that we should drink eight 8-ounce glasses of water each day, there remains no question that water is a key requirement for health. Recently published research documents that men who drink five or more 8-ounce glasses of water daily have significantly fewer heart attacks than those who drink two or fewer glasses a day. Although this same research has not yet been done for women, there is no reason to suspect the results would be any different. The reason that water consumption seems to prevent heart attacks appears to be that dehydration increases the tendency for blood to clot and, conversely, that adequate hydration prevents excess blood clotting. Blood clotting is a risk factor for heart disease that is decreased by sufficient water intake. You can see, in light of this alone, how important water is! Body weight is over half and as much as 75 percent water. Water regulates your body temperature, it helps the nutrients you take in to reach their destinations, and it helps clear byproducts in the form of waste out of the system. You can decide for yourself how much to drink in a day, but just don't forget about the importance of water!

How to Get the Nutrients You Need

Even if you don't understand the specific nutrients your body needs to function properly, you can be confident you are getting these nutrients by being sure to eat from the following dietary guidelines for daily servings from the United States Department of Agriculture:

- Two to three servings of meat, fish, eggs, beans, or nuts (one egg, one-half cup of beans, or a meat/fish portion the size of a deck of cards equals a serving);
- Two to three servings of milk, yogurt, or cheese (two ounces of cheese or one cup of milk/yogurt);
- Four to six servings of whole grains (one slice bread, one-half cup of rice/pasta, one bowl of cereal);
- Four fruit servings (one piece of fruit equals one serving);
- Five vegetable servings (one-half cup each); and
- Moderate amounts of oils and fats.

Avoid sugared cereals, canned fruit in heavy syrup, salted chips, and other prepared foods that sneak in excess salt or sugar that you don't need.

Using a Registered Dietitian

If you feel that good nutrition is the missing link in your overall health program, at some point you may decide to meet with a registered dietitian. These professionals have studied good nutrition and can save you lots of time and experimentation on your own. They are also good sources of inspiration and support. A dietitian can help you understand why your food choices are not helping, and perhaps are even hindering, your cause.

Your doctor or your local hospital can direct you to some registered dietitians (RDs) in your area. Many dietitians specialize in one area of health; cardiovascular, renal, and diabetes nutrition are common areas of specialization.

What do dietitians do? They start by getting a personal history, asking questions about your past and your current eating habits. Questions might include, have you always struggled with weight issues or is this something new? What does a typical day look like for you as far as meals and snacking? Do you eat out in restaurants a lot? Are you making meals for a family or does someone else in your family do the cooking? What kind of work do you do? What do you do about lunch during the work day? Do you eat breakfast? The dietitian then starts to educate you on the basics of good nutrition and how it applies to your specific situation, lifestyle, and health issues.

Weight Loss

Maintaining a healthy weight for your body type is considered an important aspect in managing endometriosis and, in fact, in managing almost any chronic illness. Even if excess weight itself does not contribute to worsening symptoms, eating right and exercising (and therefore weight control) are important for simply maintaining overall health. With overall good health, you strengthen your immune system and help your body better deal with things like endometriosis. Also, since fat cells facilitate estrogen use, estrogen levels increase with weight, a real issue for women with endometriosis.

Where to Begin to Lose Weight

Don't head off on some promise-you-the-moon diet. And don't try to change everything about your diet over the course of a weekend. Start with small changes—if they affect things you eat often, small changes can add up to big results. Getting to and maintaining a healthy weight is a lifelong commitment and is unique to each individual.

First, look at your everyday eating habits and tackle those. Here are some possibilities:

- Keep a food diary. Write down what and how much you put in your mouth. Many times, you'll be surprised at the amounts that you just didn't realize you were eating.

- Do you drink coffee with extra cream? Start mixing the cream with milk until, after a couple weeks, you are using only milk, preferably low-fat milk. After a month or so, you'll find cream in your coffee to be a bit repulsive! Better yet, work toward drinking coffee black or not drinking coffee at all. Do you always drink tea black? Then try making the switch to tea all together. This is not a solution if you want to get rid of caffeine, too, but if you are looking to lessen your fat intake, black tea or coffee is better than the beverage with cream or milk.

- Ditto with sugar in your coffee. Once you wean yourself from sugared coffee, you'll notice immediately if the server at your local coffee shop accidentally puts sugar in your coffee. You'll probably even return it since you'll find it so sweet as to be undrinkable!

- Do you love potato chips, nachos, or other snack items? Don't try to give them up cold turkey and set yourself up to fail. Try instead to limit your consumption. If you normally grab the whole bag and watch television or read while mindlessly reaching into the bag until it's empty, stop bringing the bag with you. Instead, take out a handful or perhaps the number of chips that is listed as a serving size on the nutrient chart. Seal the bag up, put it away, and enjoy your chips slowly. When your handful is gone, go find something else to do and keep yourself busy so you're not tempted to go back for more.

- Don't let yourself get to the point of being extremely hungry. If you can, eat something light and nutritious or not fattening every two to three hours. A piece of fruit is always good, a small bowl of healthy cereal (not the sugar-coated kind) with low-fat milk, yogurt, a handful of nuts, or a snack-sized low-fat pudding or fruit gelatin. Then when you eat a main meal you won't be so ravenous that you choose foods that counteract your attempts to diet or devour a portion much larger than you really need.

- Drink water. As mentioned earlier, there is a lot of controversy at the moment about whether eight glasses a day is really necessary. However, water is fat-free and is required for your body to function and survive, making it always a good choice. Fruit juices are often full of sugar, real unsweetened fruit juices can be expensive, diet soda is full of chemicals—why not just go for water? Plus, a glass of water can make you feel a little fuller before a meal, and you may be less tempted to eat more than an appropriate portion.

- Change your favorite things. If you love ice cream and always have a bowl in the evening, don't give it up all together and make yourself miserable. Instead, find a different favorite ice cream—look for a low-fat ice cream that you love or find a frozen yogurt flavor that is delicious and eat that instead. And make your portion in line with the serving size on the package—even use a small-sized bowl to force portion control. A common problem with low-fat food items is that people think that because the item is low in fat, you can eat as much as you want. In fact, some prepared low-fat foods are very high in sugar, something you want to cut back on when you are trying to lose weight.

- Change some food-focused habits. Do you typically go out for pizza every Friday evening with your colleagues? Do they always want to order the supreme pizza that has four different greasy meats on it and extra cheese? Then you get annoyed with yourself because you eat twice as many slices as you should because, after all, it does taste good! And, of course, pizza often means beer. Try ordering your own personal-sized pizza in a vegetarian version, no extra cheese, and eat that. Better yet, eat just half of it and bring the other half home for a quick lunch the next day. Skip the beer and order a diet soda or, better yet, a glass of water. If you don't feel you have the willpower to skip the beer or adjust your pizza intake, maybe for a while you should skip the gathering all together. Find a more healthful way to end the week and make it your new routine.

Focus on your typical "food week" and come up with your own list of six to ten things that you could easily change to start to cut back on calories and fat.

Snacking Ideas

We have been conditioned to think snacking is bad, but, like everything else, it just depends. Choosing the right snack items can actually help curb your appetite when meal times come, making it easier to stay within a good range of calorie intake at meal times.

However, if you are counting calories and fat grams, don't forget to include your snack calories in your overall count—those little chocolate-coated graham crackers can add significant calories to your day. Here are some low-calorie and low-fat snacking ideas:

- salsa with low-fat nacho chips or baked potato chips
- pita bread with tabouli
- unbuttered air-popped or microwave popcorn
- granola bars
- pretzels

- fruit (but not late at night—fruit is high in fructose, which converts to energy if you are active, but if you eat it before bedtime it will be converted to fat)
- vegetable wedges with no-fat sour cream or, better yet, salsa
- frozen yogurt or low-fat ice cream

- low-fat or fat-free yogurt. Add frozen berries or raisins to add crunch and flavor without calories

Like everything you do when it comes to losing weight, portion control is the key. A few nachos with no-fat salsa is a fine mid-afternoon snack; you just can't sit with the whole bag in front of you and snack until the jar of salsa is empty. Take a few chips out of the bag, seal it, and put it away. Dump a couple of table-spoons of salsa into a small bowl. Eat your snack slowly and enjoy it. When that portion is done, you're done. If you are more than modestly overweight, it's probably best to find a different dipper than nachos or even baked potato chips; try pretzels or crispy pita wedges.

Sources of Motivation, Support, and Discipline for Making Significant Diet and Exercise Changes

Losing weight is a difficult proposition under any circumstances. There are many ways you can combat the stress of a weight-loss program, motivate yourself to begin, and stay motivated.

1. Learn all you can about the significant benefits that people with chronic illnesses experience from weight loss. Knowledge can be a major motivator. Any time you get exasperated with your diet, thinking of these benefits can keep you going.

2. Once you've been dieting for a bit, you'll begin to lose some weight and experience some of the aforementioned benefits, which are among the strongest motivating factors. Slipping into a smaller pair of pants, reclaiming some of those favorite items in the back

of your closet, and soaking up those admiring comments from your friends can be the best motivation you can get.

3. Get some outside support. Diet with a friend—you can keep each other on track, share dieting tips, and share great diet foods and recipes. Hospitals are becoming major outlets for education, holding seminars and clinics given by professional experts. Check your local hospital for possible programs on weight loss and control. Organized, commercial weight-loss programs such as Weight Watchers and Jenny Craig are good motivators, as well.

4. Do it for yourself. Don't look at thin models and slim movie stars and put pressure on yourself to look like them or fit into some artificial measure of beauty. Many of them fully admit that they don't even look like themselves first thing in the morning! While your husband or partner will probably be the first to compliment you as you lose weight (and women who take off a few pounds often motivate overweight partners to do the same!), it is limiting and can be self-defeating to lose weight because someone else thinks you should look differently. Do it for yourself first—for your overall health, to alleviate your endometriosis symptoms, to more easily do an activity that you like to do, and to feel better about your own reflection in the mirror, too!

5. Set realistic goals. Those ads for products that help you lose "ten pounds in two days" are not only false, but encourage unhealthy weight loss. Caloric intake should be no lower than 1400 calories per day. This number combined with regular exercise should allow you to maintain a nutritious diet without being punitive. Losing

weight takes time. Stay away from the scales, but if you must weigh, plan to lose maybe three to five pounds a month for six months to a year. Give yourself time to adjust to a new way of eating, which is the key to ongoing weight control once you've lost weight, along with incorporating more exercise into your life. Once you've made some significant gains on this slow weight-loss program, maybe then step it up a notch.

6. If you go off your diet and new eating habits for an evening or even a weekend, don't despair and, most of all, don't quit! Just pick up where you left off and forget about the digression.

7. Find ways to reward yourself. Keep it simple—don't create rewards that make you feel guilty. If you are struggling with finances, don't reward yourself with expensive purchases. But if you meet a major weight goal, maybe a new scarf or a pair of earrings is a satisfying reward. If you love real ice cream, treat yourself at the local ice cream shop—but get a kid-size portion of something simple, not a huge banana split for which you are going to feel guilty. You need to celebrate!

8. Don't weigh yourself every day. Stay away from the scales if possible because this can be very discouraging; body weight can fluctuate two to three pounds per day from simple water retention without you doing anything different. Instead, if you must, pick two days of the week to weigh in, say Friday and Monday. Give yourself a range, such as staying within 140 to 145 pounds for the month of April. During those few weeks, look for ways in your

eating and exercise program to drop to the next level. Then spend a couple weeks holding under 145.

9. If a special event comes up and you suspect you will go off your diet over the weekend, you'll feel better if you are within your range on Friday. Then if Monday's weigh-in shows that you splurged enough to go above your desired range, you have the whole week to get back on track from there and compare again on Friday.

Weight loss is difficult enough. Don't put additional stress on yourself. Instead spend your energy motivating yourself, shopping for new clothes, and figuring out what you are going to do with your extra time from fewer doctor's appointments, since you will almost certainly have fewer symptoms to deal with!

Exercise

Exercising not only helps you lose weight, but weight loss also makes you feel more like exercising! Once you've shed a few pounds, you'll probably become more interested in toning your new body. Also, remember that as you convert fat to lean body mass, your weight may actually go up instead of down. This is another good reason to stay away from the scales.

Exercise is also more difficult and exhausting for someone who is overweight, and certainly for someone who doesn't exercise and is out of condition both physically and aerobically. Therefore, don't plunge into an exercise program only to wear yourself out on the first go-round. That is very discouraging.

Also, don't fall into the trap of signing up with the local fitness center and setting up a schedule of two hours four days a week doing weight lifting, the treadmill, swimming, and an aerobics class. Then you think, "there, that will do it." That will do it all right! What it will do is last maybe three weeks before you realize that there is just no way you can fit that kind of exercise program into your schedule. Even if you have all the time in the world, if you have not already been involved in a formal exercise program, you're not suddenly going to find it a great way to spend your time.

Just like with dieting, start small. Begin by looking at your day and seeing where you might fit in some changes. The following ideas have been around a long time, but they are still good ones:

- Walk more. Take the stairs, not the elevator at the office or the escalator at the mall. Park in a distant space in the parking lot and walk to the entrance of the building. Walk at lunch instead of sitting in your cubicle or hitting the drive-through at a fast-food restaurant. Go to the park with your homemade lunch and get some fresh air.

- Find something to motivate you to get outside and move around. Learn to enjoy gardening. Get a dog—there's a breed and size of dog suitable to any lifestyle, and there is nothing more motivating than a dog that needs a walk!

- Instead of using your kids as an excuse for not having time to exercise, use them to get you exercising. Hang a basketball hoop on the garage or a soccer goal or volleyball net on the lawn and play a quick game with your son or daughter before dinner. Even if your kids are still very little, bicycling can be fun for everyone.

• Go on a walk for a cause. You can find one of these going on almost every weekend. Besides getting exercise, you'll meet new people and donate to a worthy cause. If you don't want to do the entire walk, you can always just do part of it. And you can bring your kids or even the dog with you.

• Buy a few free weights for home. They aren't expensive and don't require you to find time to get to the gym. Work yourself into a gradual program of increasing repetitions (reps) and sets to tone up those arms and legs that are getting thinner as you lose weight!

Personal Trainers

If you think you don't have time to exercise regularly, then you probably don't have time to create your own successful exercise program. Consider signing on with a personal trainer. Personal trainers:

• Know a lot about nutrition and dieting and can help you learn about your own body mass index and other useful diagnostic tools for weight control
• Can teach you how to use exercise equipment, including free weights, most effectively for what you are trying to accomplish, most efficiently for your needs, and safely so that you don't hurt yourself with strains and unnecessarily sore muscles
• Can set up an exercise program tailored to you

- Are great motivators! Because their work depends on their clients, it is to their benefit that you see results.

If cost is a factor, find a personal trainer who will consider meeting with you just once a month. A concentrated amount of time at first is best so you can get lots of input on what you are doing. After that, you can maintain a certain level for a month, then check in with your trainer to make sure you are on track for your goals and to take you to the next level.

Your local YMCA or fitness center probably has personal trainers who use their facilities. Some personal trainers work from their own space, some will come to your home and some even bring their equipment with them.

Decide on a personal trainer just as you would any other professional relationship—only more so. To get the help you need, you must be very comfortable with your trainer and talk with her or him honestly and straightforwardly. You can't hide the fact that you have gone off your diet since you saw your trainer a month ago. You are the one who is getting the real benefit from this relationship, so you need to be up front with your trainer.

As with any aspect of exercise that is new to you, be sure to talk with your doctor before starting to work with a personal trainer. A professional trainer will have health documents you need to sign and have your doctor sign as well. You will also be asked to fill out a complete health and fitness history. Definitely tell your personal trainer about your endometriosis diagnosis so he or she can tailor your program with that in mind, especially working around pain issues.

What Can I Do on My Own?

Besides the day-to-day things mentioned in the previous list, what can you do to get started on a serious exercise regimen? If you are more than a few pounds overweight, start off with something to help your body be more flexible and more in tune with exercising. Plus, these kinds of programs are all great stress-reducers—and most women trying to manage endometriosis can use some help reducing stress. Here are some ideas:

> *Tai Chi*: This martial art uses slow, calculated movements to increase balance, flexibility, and awareness. Tai chi can help calm you and get you in touch with your body; it is like meditation in motion. Many fitness centers and wellness centers offer tai chi classes. Tai chi is also something fairly easy to learn and follow from a video—you can do it in the comfort of your own living room in baggy pants and an oversized T-shirt.

> *Yoga*: Yoga is not just for thin, extremely flexible people. Yoga is great for everyone—and the more you do, the more you can do! You can get videos and do yoga at home. It doesn't take a special equipment. However, it is important to be sure you are doing the positions properly to avoid injury and get the most benefit, so it is helpful to take some classes. There is also a style of yoga that is specifically intended for weight loss. These sessions move along quickly, and you don't even realize what a workout you've had until you're done!

Swimming: If you have the time and access to a good pool, swimming is a great form of exercise, especially for someone with pain issues. Your buoyancy in water takes the stress off your body, and you can exercise a little more vigorously without the impact of exercise on dry land.

Toning exercises: Some exercises take no equipment at all. Find some good exercises, such as abdominal crunches and other toning exercises, that you can do right before you shower. As with weightlifting, increase your reps and sets gradually and be patient.

Sex: It had to be mentioned. Making love is a great form of exercise. However, if your endometriosis makes sex an unappealing and painful option, of course, you'll need to take care of some of the issues related to that first. Several chapters in this book have information on pain management and intercourse-related issues.

Things to Remember While Exercising

If regular exercise has not been part of your life before now, there are some important points to keep in mind regarding exercise.

- Always talk with your primary care physician about your exercise program. That doesn't mean you shouldn't exercise until you see your doctor at your appointment six months from now. But keep it simple, build up gradually, and be sure to tell the doctor anything you are doing for exercise. If you have a specific condition—heart, lung, or muscle-related, for instance—then yes, make a special appointment to see your doctor to review your exercise plans and get a green light first.

- For any vigorous workout, drink plenty of fluids. Water is always best.

- The claim that stretching is crucial before and after exercise has come under scrutiny, but the jury is still out, so go ahead and stretch. It probably can't hurt.

- Don't overwhelm and discourage yourself, and don't try to get your exercise doing something you simply don't enjoy. It's okay not to like to swim or lift weights. To be successful and be motivated to continue, choose an exercise regimen that you don't hate.

- The old adage "no pain, no gain" is simply not true. You should not be in pain either during exercise or after. You may feel some discomfort the next day, but your muscles should not hurt in pain.

- When lifting weights, start off with a low weight size. You can always increase it if it seems too easy, but before you do that, increase the number of reps and sets first and see where you are. The idea is to have the last few reps and the last set be a little strenuous. You don't want to sideline yourself from the start by straining your muscles, and you don't want to bulk yourself up like a bodybuilder with heavy weights. And always give your muscles one day of rest between weight-lifting rounds.

- Mix it up. You don't have to get your exercise all from one activity. Some exercise routines, such as weight lifting, require repeating at least two or three times a week to see benefits. But if you want to get some aerobic exercise—and you should!—do some vigorous walking, jog, or ride a bicycle. And top it off by going dancing on Saturday night.

- Learn good posture. Not just your daily posture for sitting and standing and working at a computer, but the proper posture for the exercise you have chosen.

- Learn good breathing techniques. Most people pay little attention to their breathing, but breathing is critical for exercising well. Practicing deep, rhythmic breathing during the course of the day can be a great stress reliever. Slowly take air into your abdomen first, and then fill up your mid-chest section, then your upper chest and lungs. Exhale in the opposite way. Good breathing is simply good for you, but it is crucial while exercising.

The Ultimate Motivation

The benefits of maintaining optimum weight, eating nutritiously, and exercising are hard to overestimate when it comes to a chronic illness like endometriosis. However, don't beat yourself up if you go off your program for a couple days or things aren't moving along as quickly as you think they should. Instead, pat yourself on the back for simply getting started. Always keep in mind that endometriosis is a chronic condition that needs to be managed over time using all the tools mentioned in this book. You have the rest of your life to make progress and find out what works or what doesn't. Some people who have been diagnosed with a chronic illness admit that the diagnosis triggered them to take care of themselves, and despite the illness, they feel better than they have in years!

Endometriosis and the Food You Eat

There is nothing about your body that the food you eat does not have a connection to. Endometriosis is no exception. This importance is reflected in a quote from Susan M. Lark's booklet *Natural Treatment of Fibroid Tumors and Endometriosis*: "I cannot emphasize too strongly the importance of good dietary habits for women beginning a fibroid and endometriosis treatment program. After years of working with thousands of women patients, including many with these symptoms, I have found that no therapy can be fully effective without including beneficial dietary changes as part of the treatment plan."

The Estrogen Connection

Whether there is a connection between estrogens and endometriosis has not been discovered or documented in any reproducible study of endometriosis. There is no evidence that women who avoid soy products, for example, have fewer problems with endometriosis. There is evidence that the implants of endometriosis respond differently to hormones, and this may be part of the eventual answer to why endo symptoms are variable and frequently do not respond to treatments based on lowering estrogen levels.

The Liver's Role in Endometriosis

Some research leads to the belief that liver disorders hold a key in predisposing a woman to endometriosis. Among other important functions, the liver regulates and removes many waste chemicals from the body. If, for whatever reason, the liver begins failing to remove these wastes, symptoms such as chronic fatigue and allergies (common in endometriosis) can appear.

Studies have also shown that the liver is a major target for dioxin and is severely affected by this known toxic chemical. A significant number of people exposed to dioxin have enlarged livers and impaired liver function. Unfortunately for the liver, dioxin is present in much of the American food chain. Meat, poultry, full-fat dairy products, and certain fish account for 95 percent of dioxin exposure. Because dioxins are stored in fat, you can minimize exposure by minimizing your intake of animal fats, choosing lean cuts of meat, trimming fat, skinning poultry, and drinking low-fat milk.

Improving the liver's ability to perform its many roles vital to good health may significantly reduce endometriosis symptoms. An appropriate diet includes a high percentage of raw fruits and vegetables (organic is best), legumes (kidney beans and peas, for instance), and foods high in potassium (like bananas and raisins). Daily supplements of the herb milk thistle before meals helps the liver to maintain good function, as do several of the herbs mentioned in Chapter Seven.

Because of their high levels of vitamin B and vitamin E, whole grains also regulate hormone levels, with a beneficial effect on both the liver and the ovaries. Research has shown that B vitamin deficiency hinders the liver's ability to metabolize estrogen. Adding B vitamin supplementation to the diet of women suffering from pre-menstrual syndrome (PMS), heavy menstrual bleeding, and fibrocystic breast disease helped to decrease the severity of their symptoms. Studies conducted at UCLA Medical School during the 1980s found that taking a specific B vitamin, pyridoxine B6, helped to relieve symptoms of menstrual cramps and PMS.

Foods to Avoid

Women with endometriosis should try to avoid the following foods:

*   *Dairy*: Avoiding dairy helps to reduce pelvic pain and cramps because dairy products produce muscle-contracting F2 alpha prostaglandins. Of course, calcium is also important, so you'll need to turn to sources of calcium other than dairy products, including beans, peas, and green leafy vegetables.

    Fats: Fats also include muscle-contracting prostaglandins, and excessive amounts of fat make the liver work harder, giving it less ability to help the body keep estrogen at optimum levels.

*   *Salt*: The negative effects of salt have been well-documented. The excess fluid retention caused by too much salt intake is bad enough for all women during their menstrual period, but for women with endometriosis, salt simply exacerbates the symptoms. Even if you are conscientious about not using the salt shaker, be aware that processed foods contain high amounts of hidden salt.

    Alcohol: Drinking alcohol only in moderation or avoiding it all together just makes good sense all around. First, alcohol is high in sugar. Heavy alcohol consumption compromises liver function, which we already know is essential in helping to control endometriosis. And overuse of alcohol can cause alcohol-based nutritional deficiency, exacerbating muscle spasms, fatigue, and mood swings during your cycle.

✴ *Sugar:* Sugar's effects are the same as alcohol. And, like salt, sugar is hard to avoid in processed foods. Sugar is also addicting. Find naturally sweet things to eat or use honey. There are many new food products in most grocery stores that cater to people with diabetes who are looking to avoid simple carbohydrates, so you should have no trouble finding things you like in the no-sugar aisle.

Caffeine: Like alcohol, caffeine should either be avoided or consumed in moderation. Today's "cup" of coffee is typically a mug of coffee, which is a couple of cups. If you measured the actual size of the "cups" of coffee you drink every day, the amount of coffee (and thus, caffeine) you consume may be a lot higher than you thought! Caffeine makes hot flashes and mood swings worse. In real excess, it can inhibit iron absorption, making anemia symptoms worse.

A Lot to Think About

Wow! That's a lot of daily impact. But considering how important what and how we eat is to everything we do and how we feel, it is well worth the time to understand good nutrition. Once you get into it, it can be extremely interesting.

CHAPTER NINE ∾

Fertility Issues

Fertility issues are part of the endometriosis package for as many as 30 percent of women with the disease. The good news is that the majority of women with endometriosis—two-thirds, according to most estimates—do not experience fertility problems. If you are part of that one-third who has tried unsuccessfully to conceive, there are many avenues to take. But first we should look at what causes a woman with endometriosis to experience infertility.

Endometriosis can contribute to fertility problems in several ways. This chapter takes a brief look at how the reproductive system normally works and then looks at the ways endo can compromise fertility. Finally, I'll review some processes that may be useful for improving conception in spite of endometriosis, including assisted reproductive techniques and natural approaches that may increase the odds of conceiving.

Fertility Basics

Human females are born with a lifetime's supply of eggs. At birth, the ovaries contain about a million follicles, each a collection of fluid-filled cells surrounding an immature egg. Only about 300 to 500 of these follicles develop into mature eggs during the reproductive life span, typically between puberty and about age fifty, when the possibility of egg fertilization ends with menopause, the cessation of menstruation.

During a woman's fertile years, the hypothalamus, the pituitary gland, and the ovaries communicate through hormones to regulate the phases of the reproductive cycle. In the follicular phase before ovulation, hormonal sequences support the growth of the follicle—which is the cellular complex that surrounds and nurtures the egg in the ovary—and signal the lining of the uterus to receive a fertilized egg. During this phase, the level of estrogen produced in the ovaries is low. In response to this low level of estrogen, gonadotropin-releasing hormone (GnRH) secretion increases in the hypothalamus, stimulating the pituitary gland to release low levels of follicle-stimulating hormone (FSH). This hormone instigates the follicle ripening process in the ovaries. Several days after FSH triggers growth in the follicle, estrogen begins to be released into the bloodstream on its way to the hypothalamus. Typically, ten to twenty follicles begin to develop, and usually one reaches maturity, though occasionally two or more reach this stage. The follicles also produce estrogen, and as the eggs ripen, estrogen output increases.

To produce estrogen, the follicles require small amounts of another pituitary hormone, luteinizing hormone (LH). LH stimulates the ovary cells that surround the follicle to manufacture testosterone, which is then transported to the inside of the follicle and converted to estrogen. This action signals the uterine lining (endometrium) to thicken in preparation for the possibility of nurturing a fertilized egg. This is the beginning of the second menstrual phase, proliferation.

By now, one follicle has become dominant and produces rapidly increasing amounts of estrogen. Some of this hormone secretion is bound to a protein in the bloodstream known as sex-hormone binding globulin (SHBG). During their reproductive years, women have double the concentration of SHBG that men have, because estrogens encourage SHBG production. Androgens, such as testosterone, suppress SHBG production.

The hormones captured by SHBG become basically inert. The production of cervical mucus begins. FSH production declines, removing support from the competing lesser follicles. Declining FSH levels also make the dominant follicle receptive to LH. When the estrogen levels are sufficient around the middle of the cycle and the egg approaches maturity, the follicle releases a burst of progesterone. In response, GnRH increases, signaling the pituitary gland to secrete large amounts of both FSH and LH. Within 36 hours of this surge, the now-mature follicle bursts, releasing the egg (ovulation). This is the optimum time for fertilization of the egg by male sperm.

After Ovulation

At ovulation, the follicle and the ovarian surface open over the egg. The egg is released and picked up by the finger-like tendrils of the fallopian tube. The fallopian tube itself is highly flexible muscular structure capable of precisely coordinated movement. If a woman has sexual intercourse during this fertile time, the egg and the sperm meet in the outer half of the fallopian tube.

Under the influence of LH, the now-empty follicle is transformed in function and becomes known as the corpus luteum. It will take over from the hypothalamus and release both estrogen and progesterone during the proliferation phase of the cycle.

In response to the progesterone increase from the follicle, the thickening uterine lining begins to secrete nutrients in preparation for receiving a fertilized egg. A fertilized egg can only implant during this nourishing phase, which can last from six to twenty days. If fertilization occurs, these nutrients sustain a growing embryo until the placenta develops and the mother's blood supply can nourish the fetus during the rest of the pregnancy.

The Final Luteal Phase

A woman ovulates once a cycle. The egg lives twelve to twenty-four hours and then disintegrates if not fertilized. In favorable cervical mucus conditions (cervical mucus nourishes and guides the sperm, which would otherwise die in about a half-hour or never reach the egg), sperm can survive as long as five days within the body. If the mature egg is fertilized, the corpus luteum then provides the estrogens and progesterone necessary to sustain the pregnancy until the placenta takes over this job at about 10 weeks' gestation.

How Fertility May be Restricted

Although the pregnancy rates for women with endometriosis remain slightly lower than those of the general population, most do not experience fertility problems. However, severe endometriosis is considered one of the three major causes of female infertility. Although how this happens is not fully understood, endometriosis may result in failure to ovulate (17 percent), cause a luteal phase defect that interferes with implantation, or cause a luteinized unruptured follicle (LUF) in which eggs ripen but do not release from the follicle.

How minimal endometriosis affects fertility is still not clear, though previously undiagnosed endo is commonly discovered during laparoscopic investigation among women being treated for infertility. It is hypothesized that the prostaglandins (hormones) secreted by active, newer endometrial implants may interfere with the reproductive organs by causing muscular contractions or spasms. Because there is an increased volume of peritoneal fluid (fluid in the abdominal/pelvicregion) with endometriosis, peritoneal macrophages (scavenger white blood cells) increase in both number and activity. Under this chemical influence, the fallopian tube may be unable to pick up the egg. Also, the stimulated uterus may reject implantation. In addition, sperm motility and the ability of the sperm to penetrate into the egg may be adversely affected by increased peritoneal fluid.

However, the good news is that often the reproductive organs remain functional. For a woman with mild endo whose partner has normal sperm, the statistical likelihood of conceiving is over 80 percent. If after a year of unprotected sex you haven't yet conceived despite the friendlier statistics for mild endo, you may want to consider assisted reproductive technologies or complementary approaches, which are discussed later in the chapter.

Getting pregnant may prove more of a challenge in the presence of the pronounced endometrial growth characteristic of advanced endo. Chronic tissue inflammation leads to the formation of adhesions and scars, which surround and entrap delicate reproductive organs. As the disease spreads, the older endometrial cells die out, leaving scar tissue in their wake that may block the fallopian tubes or fix them in place so that the projections on the tubes (cilia) can't grasp the egg and move it into the tube. Scarring from endometriosis may obstruct the fallopian tubes so that if an egg is fertilized, it may be unable to travel to the uterus for implantation. This type of scarring occurs only in severe endo, and interestingly, the fallopian tubes are frequently spared despite very severe disease. Many women make it well into their third decade before endometriosis is diagnosed because they were symptom free (no pain) and conceived without difficulty.

Endometrial tissue may cover part of one or both ovaries and interfere with the release of ripened eggs. The eggs themselves can be trapped in the heavy scar tissue surrounding the ovaries. In addition, the bleeding associated with endometrial cells may cause a blood-filled cyst known as an endometrioma to form over one or both ovaries. This cyst is commonly referred to as a chocolate cyst due to the brown color of accumulated blood. In women with severe pelvic adhesions where the ovary is encased, LUF may be a factor. This is believed to occur when, despite normal hormonal parameters (LH surge), the egg is not released from the ovary.

Protein Deficiencies Linked to Infertility

Clinical studies have recently identified two proteins that are missing in some women with endometriosis. Normally present in the lining of the uterus between days twenty and twenty-eight of the menstrual cycle, these proteins, beta-3 and leukemia inhibitory factor, are thought to allow the embryo to adhere to the endometrium. The absence of these proteins may account for an inability to implant an embryo or carry a fetus to term.

Treatment with GnRH drugs has been helpful in correcting beta-3 deficiencies. Some researchers think that testing for this deficiency allows women and their doctors to remedy the imbalance before beginning costly and stressful reproductive procedures, which may not succeed until this is corrected. This deficiency, however, has not been directly linked to fertility problems and should not be considered an absolute in fertility considerations.

Conception Considerations

For some women with endometriosis, the decision of whether to try to conceive now or sometime in the future may add another layer of complication to a life that's probably already quite complex. Hormonal endometriosis treatments that improve day-to-day well-being could compromise future chances for a successful pregnancy; after all, their goal, in some cases, is to deprive the body of estrogen, without which there can be no fertilization. Surgery to remove endo implants may lead to adhesions that thwart the future meeting of egg and sperm. Fertility drugs, which are typically used to increase the odds of conception, in all likelihood exacerbate endometriosis. If a genetic link for endo is proven, the possibility of passing this disease on to a daughter or granddaughter may cause some heartache, too. Quality of life may be an important factor to weigh when deciding whether to add the inevitable life stresses of raising children, especially if endo symptoms are debilitating; after all, pregnancy is only the first step in parenting, which is a lifetime commitment. There's a lot to consider.

Many women are certain that they want to experience pregnancy and raise a child, maybe more than one, despite the presence of endo. If their disease is mild or moderate, they may decide to choose treatments that preserve chances of future conception. They may choose to avoid hormonal or surgical treatments and adopt a policy of monitoring endo progress, or they may explore natural therapies. If endometriosis is advanced, becoming pregnant may be more difficult. These women may opt for more aggressive fertility treatments to overcome the physical liabilities to conception that endo may present.

A Respite from Endo?

Women with endometriosis report that their period-related endo symptoms were minimized during pregnancy—although symptoms usually reappear within a year after birth, so it's important to understand that pregnancy isn't a cure. Breast-feeding, which suppresses ovulation, tends to delay the return of endo symptoms, which makes sense because hormonal changes are at the heart of the pregnancy respite.

There are three types of estrogen produced by the body: estradiol, estrone, and estriol. Estradiol, produced by the ovaries during a menstrual cycle, strongly stimulates endometriosis to grow. When the other two types of estrogen, estrone and estriol, are present, they can fill the estrogen receptor that estradiol seeks, weakly stimulate it, and block out estradiol. Estriol is available in greater quantities during pregnancy because the fetal adrenal glands produce precursors to estriol and the placenta contributes several times the estriol normally available.

Progesterone—pro means for and gesterone means gestation—is also produced by the placenta during pregnancy. Progesterone signals the ovary to stop ovulating and maintains the spongy quality of the uterus needed from pregnancy through birth. Levels of progesterone increase dramatically throughout pregnancy. During regular menstrual cycles, a woman produces 20 mg per day of progesterone. During the peak of pregnancy, the woman's body produces 400 mg per day of progesterone. Following birth, progesterone levels drop abruptly in preparation for resuming the menstrual cycle.

Timing Matters

Whatever the stage and severity of endometriosis, a common denominator for successful conception is timing. One of the many gray areas in understanding endo is whether the disease is universally progressive. Clearly for some women, it is. Even if lesions don't proliferate, quality of life may be affected if symptoms increase over time. So if you want to conceive and it's a good time in your life to do so, most endometriosis experts would advise that pregnancy not be postponed. If the disease worsens, so do your odds of carrying a pregnancy to term.

Weigh your options carefully to avoid feeling pressured into pregnancy, though. I'm astounded by the number of very young single women who have been advised by physicians that they should become pregnant right away because of their endometriosis. Many women report anger and frustration that stem from a feeling of loss of control over decisions about child-bearing that not only endometriosis but also their doctor seems to impose. Unresolved stresses related to decisions about childbirth and pregnancy can reappear as postpartum depression, according to some studies. Fertility issues may be among the most emotionally charged in your life, but a careful review of all options now, including adoption, could be your best insurance for peace of mind.

Also factor in post-surgical timing issues. Pregnancy rates are highest during the first six months to a year after conservative endo surgery, which corrects mechanical and structural abnormalities and drains peritoneal fluid. After that brief window of opportunity, any endo left behind may flare and create additional inflammation and scarring. Chances of conceiving after such surgery may be higher than with in vitro fertilization. Surgical interventions for endometriosis are discussed in detail in Chapter Four.

If hormone drugs, such as birth control pills, have been used to control endo, be sure to wait the time period recommended by your doctor— at least one normal menstrual cycle—after treatment has stopped to try to get pregnant. And because some long-acting progesterone therapies may suppress ovulation for as long as a year after treatment ceases, don't choose this therapy if pregnancy is desired.

What's the best way to maximize the window of opportunity after surgery? If your disease is mild, you are under 35, and have no additional fertility issues, try to figure out when you are most likely to ovulate, perhaps using a basal body temperature thermometer (temperature will increase a fraction after ovulation) or an ovulation prediction kit (which measures hormones in urine), and use the results to time intercourse to coincide with the release of an egg. There are seven days in a cycle when conception is possible: five days before an egg is released (because sperm can survive for five days) and two days after ovulation, after which the egg will be shed. If you haven't conceived after six months to a year of unprotected sex, it may be time to seek help from fertility specialists.

If your endometriosis is more advanced or you want to maximize your chances of becoming pregnant despite the risks of drugs or surgery, you may want to proceed directly to assisted reproductive techniques. Surgical therapy may offer the best means of pregnancy for most women with endo because surgery has no drug effects that can compromise trying to conceive. However, many women may wish to postpone this decision and may be well served with symptom reduction based on medical therapy.

What to Expect from Fertility Consultations

Try to schedule your first consultation with a fertility specialist (called reproductive endocrinologists) during the first week of your cycle, counting from the first day of menstruation. Keep track of the length of your menstrual cycles for several months beforehand. Charting basal body temperatures (BBTs) for several months will also give your doctor some insights, as will recording the results from home ovulation predictor tests. BBTs can be a bit problematic and are fraught with some irregularities that are frustrating in an already difficult situation. Baseline blood tests for FSH and LH must be done on day three of your cycle. If your consultation should take place before that, you'll be instructed to come in for these tests on day three of your cycle.

Additional tests may be conducted on the day of LH surge (mid-cycle) and again about seven days after ovulation.

At the first appointment, most reproductive endocrinologists also do routine screening of both partners for AIDS, hepatitis, etc. A semen analysis for your partner will be scheduled. Medical histories for both partners will be taken. Some doctors accept your medical records for review before your appointment. If not, bring your medical records with you.

Another appointment should be scheduled before ovulation, on the day of the LH surge. In most cases, you will be directed to use home ovulation test kits and call for an appointment on the day you detect a surge. Included in this exam are the following tests:

Cervical mucus tests: These include a post-coital test (PCT) to test whether the sperm can penetrate and survive in the cervical mucus, plus a bacterial screening. It is important to note that the appropriate time to do PCTs is just before ovulation, around the time of the LH surge, when mucus is the most receptive. PCTs at other times may give false results.

Ultrasound exam: On the day of the LH surge, ultrasound is used to assess the thickness of the endometrium (lining of the uterus), monitor follicle development, and assess the condition of the uterus and ovaries. A thin lining indicates a hormonal problem. Many doctors order a second ultrasound two or three days after the first. This second ultrasound confirms that the follicle actually did release the egg and can rule out LUF syndrome, a situation in which eggs ripen but do not release from the follicle.

Further testing may include a hysterosalpingogram (HSG). The HSG determines whether the uterine cavity is normal in shape and if the fallopian tubes are open. If this test is warranted, a specialist injects dye through the cervix into the uterus and takes a series of x-ray pictures as the dye flows through the fallopian tubes and outlines the female reproductive tract. The HSG can detect uterine fibroids, polyps, and obstructions in one or both of the fallopian tubes. This test is performed after a menstrual period but before anticipated ovulation.

Based on the findings of these examinations, you and your doctor can formulate a plan to determine which assisted reproductive techniques may best enhance your chances of conception.

Assisted Reproductive Techniques
Intrauterine Insemination
Generally considered the least invasive fertility enhancement approach, intrauterine insemination (IUI) involves charting your ovulation cycles to predict when an egg will be released. When fertility is likely, a doctor injects concentrated sperm from your partner or a donor into your uterus. The procedure doesn't exacerbate endometrial growth or scarring.

As long as your fallopian tubes and ovaries are intact, ovarian stimulation may be combined with IUI. Ovulation-induction medications, often referred to as fertility drugs, are used to stimulate the follicles in your ovaries. The medications also control the time that you release the eggs, or ovulate, so sexual intercourse, IUIs, and in vitro fertilization procedures can be scheduled at the most likely time to achieve pregnancy. GnRH drugs may be used to control and predict egg maturation. Some medications stimulate ovary production (Clomid); others stimulate production of multiple eggs in a single cycle. However, these hormones can boost estrogen production to levels that can stimulate endometrial flare-ups and growth, including cyst formation, so your doctor may recommend limiting the use of such drugs to six cycles or fewer. Natural-cycle procedures, where a single egg is harvested and then implanted, may be worth considering. Ultrasound is usually used extensively during these treatments to assess the activity of the ovaries and the endometrial lining, so be prepared for this test to be repeated sometimes daily.

In Vitro Fertilization Techniques

Gamete intrafallopian transfer (GIFT) combines fertility drugs with laparoscopy. A surgeon removes ripe eggs from the ovaries and immediately places them in your fallopian tubes along with sperm. In another approach, zygote intrafallopian transfer (ZIFT), a surgeon retrieves eggs transvaginally, using an ultrasound probe to guide a hollow needle into the ovaries to aspirate eggs, which are then combined with sperm in a dish. The resulting zygotes are then placed in the fallopian tubes, where they can travel on their own into the uterus, with increased odds of pregnancy.

In IVF (in vitro fertilization), the fertilization of eggs also occurs outside of the female body, in a Petri dish. Using a needle guided by ultrasound to remove multiple eggs from the woman's ovary, doctors then combine the eggs with sperm. The resulting embryos are kept in an incubator for several days and allowed to divide and multiply. The developing embryos are then placed into the uterus via a thin plastic catheter that's introduced through the cervix. Success rates vary, and you should ask about live birth rates, as opposed to pregnancy statistics, when considering this procedure.

Ectopic Pregnancy

Women with endometriosis may have a higher rate of ectopic pregnancy (estimated to be sixteen times more likely than in women without endometriosis), a potentially life-threatening condition in which the fertilized egg implants and begins to develop outside the uterus.

The most frequent sites for abnormal implantation are the fallopian tubes. Rarely, the egg implants in the cervix, in one of the two ovaries, or in the abdominal cavity. The warning signs of tubal ectopic pregnancy are pelvic cramping that is low and to one side, shoulder pain, dizziness, and vaginal spotting beginning shortly after the first missed menstrual period.

Occasionally, an ectopic pregnancy is absorbed by the body. However, if growth exceeds the capacity of the tube to expand, the tube may rupture. This can cause many serious problems, including bleeding, infection, infertility, or even death. Therefore, early diagnosis and assessment are critical in determining the appropriate care to maintain your safety and health.

Doctors can measure the levels of progesterone in the blood to assist in the diagnosis of abnormal pregnancies. If tests indicate that you have an ectopic pregnancy, surgery is the most likely scenario. Doctors will begin surgery as soon as possible to minimize danger to your health.

Natural Approaches to Fertility

Because natural therapies focus on restoring balance to both the physical and energetic systems of the body, they can be of value to women with endometriosis who have problems conceiving. In general, if scarring and other physical blockage issues exist, surgical correction of these problems may be advisable. Consult with an experienced practitioner before beginning on a balancing program to get maximum benefit from natural fertility approaches.

Avoid Nicotine

In England, researchers reported that smoking diminishes fertilization in women by two-thirds. A study by the University of Bristol and St. George's Hospital Medical School revealed that cotinine, the main by-product of nicotine, is a long-lasting substance that concentrates in the follicular fluid of the ovaries and affects conception.

Herbal Fertility Support

Because the liver is the most important organ for estrogen removal and hormone regulation, liver health can affect fertility. To strengthen and rebuild the liver, drink teas made from black cohosh, goldenseal, and red clover. (You can brew tea from one herb at a time or combine two or three.) Burdock helps eliminate toxins from the liver, and chicory, milk thistle, and dandelion root stimulate and cleanse the liver.

Black cohosh and vitex (chaste tree berry): These herbs naturally assist in the releasing of LH by stimulating the pituitary gland in the brain. These supplements are known for regulating ovulation and for helping those with amenorrhea (absent menstrual periods). Women who are prescribed Clomid may want to consider taking both of these natural cycle regulators.

Blue cohosh (Caulophyllum thalictroides): Blue cohosh comes from an entirely different genus than black cohosh. It is a uterine tonic, meaning it can relax a hypersensitive uterus as well as increase the muscular tone of a weak uterus. Early American herbal guides list blue cohosh as a uterine botanical helpful in cases of infertility.

Nutritional Support

For men and women, a nutritious diet supplemented with a multivitamin and free of hormones and pesticides goes a long way toward improving both reproductive and overall health. Dietary sources of estrogens may play some role in infertility, especially when the liver is already stressed. Both dairy products and meat (especially animal fat) have estrogen content. Pesticide sprays (xenoestrogens) also contribute to our estrogen intakes. In addition, many herbs and foods have estrogenic activities. It is advisable for women with infertility problems to monitor their diet and minimize estrogen intake.

Selenium deficiencies have been linked to infertility in both men and women. Since selenium levels vary among geographic areas, the food we eat that usually provides this mineral (such as broccoli, red grapes, garlic, and onions) can no longer be relied on to provide adequate levels. The recommended level of supplementary selenium is 200 mcg daily.

Para-aminobenzoic acid (PABA) stimulates the pituitary gland and can restore fertility to some infertile women.

Homeopathy Might Help

Because homeopathic medicines can be effective in reestablishing health in women's reproductive organs, they can also be helpful in reestablishing fertility. Homeopathic constitutional care, rather than self-care, is necessary for treating fertility problems, so consult with an experienced homeopathic practitioner to develop a program to improve fertility.

Chinese/Oriental Medicine

Both acupuncture and Chinese herbs have strong track records for helping women who have experienced trouble becoming pregnant to conceive. Oriental medicine for women can regulate hormones, stimulate ovulation, and correct nutritional deficiencies that make sustaining a pregnancy difficult. The herbs help create a more hospitable environment for conception, and the treatment is effective and gentle. However, for women with a structural problem such as blocked tubes, traditional Chinese medicine may not be enough to overcome blockages; IVF may be advised.

Until recently, women have had no proven method to improve their odds with each IVF attempt. The first significant scientific proof that acupuncture can improve pregnancy rates in cases of structural fertility problems has recently resulted from a well-designed German study on acupuncture-assisted reproduction therapy. The 160 participants were divided into two groups, each receiving a standard in vitro procedure (IVF). One of the groups, however, received acupuncture before and after implantation. The standard in vitro group had a 26.3 percent pregnancy rate, while the acupuncture group showed a 42.5 percent success rate. Combining Oriental and Western medical techniques may be a valid approach to overcoming infertility when reproductive structures have been damaged by endo.

Massage Releases Adhesions

An article appearing in the December 1998 issue of *Natural Health* magazine entitled, "Massage Delivers Babies," focuses on an alternative, non-surgical soft tissue myofascial release technique that has been effective in treating women with infertility problems related to adhesions and scarring. Forty percent of all female infertility is attributed to scarring, pelvic adhesions, or tubal obstruction. In myofascial release, a deep-tissue massage technique is used to slowly stretch and break up scar tissue caused by inflammation, infection, surgery, or trauma. Results from early pilot studies indicate a 50 percent full-term pregnancy rate for infertile women who were accepted into the Wurn Technique program in Gainesville, Florida (the focus of the article).

According to the web site www.clearpassage.com, adhesions and cross-links may connect the injured tissues to nerves (causing pain) or to neighboring structures (causing dysfunction). As tissues heal and adhesions form, the tissues shrink somewhat, resulting in restricted mobility in the injured area, creating more irritation and more cross-linking of collagen fibers, and perpetuating the cycle of adhesion formation. The primary goal of myofascial release therapy is to increase mobility (motion) and decrease pain using specific techniques to break down the excess cross-links at the core of adhesion formation. It is important to note here that there is no scientific proof of either improved fertility rates or pain reduction from this type of therapy.

It's Your Choice

How you choose to approach infertility problems is a very personal decision. Many factors need to be weighed, including the emotional and stress-related ones. But certainly women with endometriosis should be comforted by the fact that they most likely can conceive despite endometriosis (barring other fertility issues). It may take a lot of investigation and experimentation, but nothing worth having has ever come easy!

A PERSONAL STORY

Carrie

Carrie was 26 years old when she first had an inkling that something was going on with her body. Although she had always had normal menstrual cycles, she began to have some break-through bleeding between periods. A month or so after that began, she had stomach pain right before starting her period. Later that year, her symptoms had escalated to the point that she had severe pain two to three days before her period began and on the first day of her period.

"It was the most intense pain I ever felt," Carrie said. "I've broken bones before, but this was no comparison."

Carrie realized that her symptoms were somehow related to her period. She went to her OB/GYN, who she had seen for several years. Carrie had never complained about her health, so when the doctor pressed on her ovaries and the pain was so bad Carrie started crying, her doctor had no trouble taking her seriously.

Their first move was to put Carrie on tri-phasal birth control pills. Although it did help, the birth control made her "pretty crazy," she said. "My periods were a lot less painful, but I felt horrible." So she went off the pills. But the pain was bad— even walking downstairs was excruciating.

Every three months Carrie had an ultrasound of her ovaries, which always showed the lesions getting worse. She reviewed the findings with her doctor, and they decided to schedule laparoscopic surgery. The surgery, done in February of 2002, revealed two large lesions on her ovaries. Her doctor was appalled with the extent of the lesions. Although Carrie felt that she was being taken seriously all along, she describes the doctor as totally sympathetic with her situation after what he saw in the surgery.

After the laparoscopy, Carrie went on monophasic birth control pills, making her body think it is always in the second phase of the menstrual cycle, where no endometrium buildup takes place. And she feels, finally, just great.

"I can now go out with confidence and not worry about whether I'll end up in excruciating pain." She explains that as an avid Dave Matthews fan, she knew her endometriosis was taking control when it kept her from attending his concert. No more!

Like most women who have endured a long haul to work through this life-controlling medical problem, Carrie definitely has advice for other women struggling either with endometriosis or with some problem that is as-yet undefined:

"You only have one body. Trust it. It's giving you signs that something is wrong, trust those signs. Don't ignore them. And when you start to seek help, don't take 'no' for an answer."

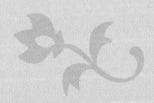

CHAPTER TEN ∾

A Winning Health Care Team
Working With Your Doctor, Medical Specialists,
and Other Team Members

If you suspect you have endometriosis—or if a diagnosis has already been confirmed—the quality of your relationship with your doctor (or doctors) will have a profound effect on your well-being. Women with endometriosis who report satisfaction with their care say that having a compassionate, communicative doctor and learning as much as they could about the disease were key factors in their adjustment to living with endo.

Because endometriosis affects each woman differently, it is essential to establish clear, honest communication with your doctor. The single truth about endometriosis is that there are no clear-cut, universal answers. If you want to have a child, that will have a bearing on your treatment plan. If pregnancy is not an issue, your treatment decisions will probably depend primarily on the severity of symptoms and differ from the decisions of someone who is concerned mainly with fertility. Decisions about endometriosis treatment can be difficult and confusing. Make it a goal to become a partner with your primary care physician so you can arrive at the best treatment decisions possible—together.

Perhaps you already have a primary care physician who doubles as your gynecologist. Perhaps your gynecologist is the only doctor you see regularly. For women with healthy reproductive systems, one doctor may fit the bill for routine care. However, if you have moderate to severe endometriosis symptoms and hormonal or surgical care is required, you should find a doctor for your team who is experienced specifically in the care and treatment of endo. Many times, women are referred to a reproductive endocrinologist (RE, a gynecologic sub-specialist in fertility problems). An RE may not be the best choice for you, because many if not most REs are in vitro fertilization specialists who are not the best alternative for endo, particularly if surgery is considered the best solution.

Other members of your health care team may include a dietitian to help with the nutritional aspects of good health in general and endometriosis in particular. You may have a naturopath to help you with alternative approaches to endometriosis treatment or specific symptoms. Or you may work with an alternative care specialist, such as a massage therapist, chiropractor, or acupuncturist.

The important thing to keep in mind is that although the team is composed of experts who know more about their chosen field of expertise than you do, you are the team captain. It may seem like a lot of work to captain a group of individuals who will probably never be in the same room together—and it is a lot of work! But it can also be very rewarding. With the knowledge you have obtained and the cooperation of your team members, endo can be under your control. When you start to get control of your endometriosis, your symptoms subside, and the focus of your world begins to change direction from being controlled by endometriosis to controlling it, you'll be proud of your perseverance!

Why an Endometriosis Specialist?

Statistics show nine years to be the average lag between the onset of endo symptoms and the definitive diagnosis of endometriosis. As I've noted, endometriosis symptoms can mimic many other conditions. When you talk or correspond over the Internet with other women who have endo, the themes of delayed diagnosis, misdiagnosis, and/or failure to excise lesions at all or completely will probably come up. Often, many doctors, including gynecologists, aren't as informed about the various manifestations and symptoms of endometriosis as you might hope, which contributes to delayed diagnosis and treatment. It is a complex condition that can be elusive.

Because an endometriosis diagnosis can only be confirmed via laparoscopy (including tissue biopsy if visual confirmation is unclear), your endo care team will likely include a surgeon. Managing the disease with an endo expert who is both skilled and experienced enough to locate and thoroughly remove endo (excision) from the beginning may prevent unnecessary repeat surgeries and ineffective treatment measures.

Endometriosis specialists are in practice solely to treat endo and pelvic pain. They do not practice routine gynecology or deliver babies. Surgeons typically perform dozens of endo procedures in a month and are skilled both in recognizing the different types of endo and in using the delicate surgical techniques required to excise endo in all its forms. And after so many surgeries, they become skilled in recognizing some of the more elusive traits of endometriosis. Also, these experts may already have ancillary help, such as bowel surgeons, urologists, or pain management experts, that can facilitate your care.

Reproductive Endocrinologist (RE)

Depending on your situation, an RE may be another specialist who can help manage endometriosis, especially if infertility is the focus of your attack on endometriosis. Endocrinologists work primarily through prescribing hormone medications. REs are physicians who received formal obstetrics and gynecology sub-specialty training in the field of hormonal regulation of reproduction and the treatment of infertility. The goals of medical treatment of endometriosis are to control progression of the disease through hormone regulation and to relieve pain and enhance fertility for women who want to conceive now or in the future. Hormone therapy may be prescribed along with conservative surgery. (Chapter Three discusses drug treatment for endo, and Chapter Nine explores fertility issues related to women with endo.)

Historically speaking, REs were first associated with laparoscopy, which is the main surgical method of treating endometriosis, so endo patients were initially referred to REs. Also, because endo was associated with infertility, REs were the recipient of these patients. However, because endometriosis-related infertility is predominately a surgical problem and because operative laparoscopy is the bailiwick of the pelvic surgeon, the RE may not be the very best alternative. So be careful to check it out carefully. It's your body and you are in control.

Later in the chapter, issues surrounding care for autoimmune conditions that commonly coincide with an endometriosis diagnosis are also explored. First, let's look at working with your doctor to treat endo.

Finding a Qualified Surgeon

If you're looking for long-term relief from endometriosis and the pain it brings, surgery with an endo specialist is something you should consider. Conservative surgery seeks to remove or destroy the growths, relieve pain, and perhaps allow future pregnancy, if desired. The least invasive kind of surgery, and therefore the most preferred, is laparoscopy (an outpatient surgery in which the surgeon views the inside of the abdomen through a tiny lighted tube inserted through one or more small abdominal incisions). A laparotomy (a more extensive procedure that requires a larger bikini-line incision and a longer recovery period) may be warranted if, for example, other organs have been invaded by endometriosis. Radical surgery, which may be advisable in severe cases, involves hysterectomy, removal of all growths, and, rarely, removal of ovaries. This type of radical surgery is rarely required. (See

Chapter Four to learn more about surgical options.) Although surgery is not considered a cure, when done by an expert surgeon, it can often provide relief for many years.

So how do you find a qualified surgeon? Contact support groups in your community, get in touch with endo organizations like the Endometriosis Association or the Endometriosis Research Center for referrals, search Internet message board communities for positive references, and call your local hospital, state medical board, or the American Medical Association to locate specialists. Often, the most reliable endo doctor referrals arrive by word of mouth. Talk to other women with endometriosis and find out who their doctors are, what experiences they've had, and whether they would recommend a particular physician. Although endometriosis treatment is a relatively recent area of specialization, there is a slowly growing number of specialists across the country—and around the world.

Help Your Doctor Help You

A common report from women is that their primary care doctors and gynecologists fail to take their symptoms seriously, at least initially. Often the pain-specific symptoms of endometriosis are determined to be the normal course of a woman's monthly cycle or other "women's issues." Because some doctors may adopt a "wait and see" attitude at first, return for another appointment if you think this doctor might help you if he/she understood your situation more fully. Prepare for the consultation beforehand. You want to present your case succinctly and convincingly with the goals of having your physician take your complaints seriously and of you playing an active role in your own health care. If you sit back passively and let the doctor tell you what you are feeling, it may be a long time before you get to the phase where treatment can actually help.

Organize a written list of your symptoms, including frequency, previous treatment, and any other relevant information. You can read from the list if you like and leave a copy for the doctor to review.

When you schedule the appointment, request a longer consultation to be sure you have enough time to fully discuss your situation and learn all you can about options.

Take notes, and ask for explanations of anything you don't understand. Ask again if necessary. If your doctor allows it, use a small tape recorder to record your conversation so you can have the information you need to do further research and find answers to your questions. (However, never tape any conversation without first getting the permission of the person you will be taping.)

Bring someone along for support and to help you remember what the doctor says.

Be as clear and assertive as you can (this is why having a list of questions in hand can be particularly helpful) and expect your doctor to listen and focus on you. Keep in mind that both doctor and patient are only human, but be sure that the doctor is willing (indeed, welcomes the idea) to work with you in a partnership. If not, it would be best to find another doctor.

For a doctor you're considering who is not yet your current doctor, first find out the basics, such as whether the doctor is accepting new patients and whether the office is open during hours that are convenient for you. Then, the following questions related to delivery of your care may be worth exploring:

- How long have you been in practice?
- Are you board-certified (by the American Board of Obstetrics and Gynecology)?
- What billing arrangements do you accept?
- Does the office file insurance claims for patients?
- At which hospitals do you have surgery privileges? Who will be doing the billing in these instances?
- If I call the office with a medical question, can I speak directly to you?
- Who do I see if you are on vacation?
- How long is the wait for appointments? Is it possible to be seen within two or three days of my call—or is it typically a one- or two-month wait?
- How do you feel about second opinions?
- How willing are you to refer me to another specialist, if need be?
- Are you associated with a hospital or medical clinic?
- Do you have admitting privileges at the hospital I prefer?

If you are considering integrating any complementary therapies into your endometriosis protocol, this might be a good time to inquire whether this physician is supportive and/or knowledgeable about natural choices in endo care.

If you have a sense that this doctor isn't a good match for you, trust your instincts, say thank you, and find another doctor. If you are comfortable and confident in this doctor's ability to work with you in treating your disease, proceed to the next step: learn more about your doctor's specific history with endometriosis treatment.

Learn About Your Doctor's Capabilities

When selecting a physician or specialist, learn all you can about his/her capabilities in treating endometriosis. Be aware that much of the success of surgical procedures relies on the experience of the surgeon. Refer to Chapter Four for information about the surgical options available. Here are some questions you may want to ask during the initial appointment.

- How many women with endometriosis do you treat? How familiar are you with the disease?
- How do you keep on top of current knowledge regarding endometriosis?
- Is obstetrics a large proportion of your practice? (Note: This information may help determine the odds of whether or not—and how frequently—your doctor may have to leave for the delivery room during your appointment. You can ask that questions specifically as well.)
- How do you determine the proper course of treatment?
- What approach do you prefer to control the occurrence of chronic pain?
- What surgical method do you perform to remove lesions? (Note: If this doctor prefers options you'd rather avoid [such as

cauterization or ablation, perhaps], then select another doctor who is skilled in preferred surgical techniques.)

- How much experience do you have with laparoscopies, laparotomies, and hysterectomies?
- Do you have colleagues available to consult during surgery in the event that the disease presents itself in an area or organ outside of your expertise?
- Will the tissues you surgically remove be sent to pathology for final identification? (Remember, unless a pathologist microscopically examines the tissues removed, it is difficult to be certain if endometriosis is present.)
- What measures do you take to reduce the chance that adhesions will form after surgery?
- Will I have ready access to all of my medical records?

The Managed Care Referral Process

Managed care as we know it in the United States today is not the friend of the patient or the physicians trying to provide care for the patient. Managed care has always been a method of individuals other than the providers of medical care to attempt to keep a portion of the health care dollar without allowing it to go toward the patient's well-being. There certainly is a place for a strong primary-care referral system with highly trained specialists who have the expertise to solve patients' problems with minimal illness and increased efficiency, resulting in lower costs. However, managed care today recruits the cheapest doctors and clinics by promising more and more volume to these needy caregivers. This results in an overburdened system in which physicians have little time to spend with patients and little incentive to do an excellent job. Overall, therefore, poorer care is delivered in volume while the best specialty care is forced to work outside this highly inefficient, yet extremely costly system.

Most of the endometriosis specialists that I am familiar with, therefore, cannot be easily accessed through typical managed care plans. This does not mean that you cannot use their services, but you may have to try a little harder to see them. Most plans have a clause that states that if a specific treatment is not available within the plan then it must be paid for outside of the plan. If the doctor that you want to see is not on your plan, check for this option and keep trying. Write letters, make phone calls, and be sure to write down names and dates to document your efforts. Generally speaking, plans don't want to evade payment—they just want to delay payment as long as possible. Plan managers figure that if they can delay sufficiently, a percentage of patients will give up and pay the costs themselves or the plan may be able to force the provider to accept a lower reimbursement. If nothing else, if the plan delays payment for a long period of time, then at least it has held the money for a period of time and made money on the interest.

This all sounds a little cynical, but in my experience as a physician who always wants to provide an extremely high level of care to his patients, this managed care alphabet soup (HMO, PPO, IPA, etc.) attempts to defeat such goals. I want my patients—and all patients, for that matter—to have access to and to receive the absolute best health care available. To do this, I think patients need to take charge of their own health care and become the "consumer" of this care. Where possible, become an active member of committees making health insurance choices at your workplace or make a choice to have your own health insurance. It just makes very little sense to try to sell wellness at bargain or discount prices and still expect the extraordinary level of care that Americans have become accustomed to.

Take charge of this area of your wellness, too. You can make a difference with education and the help of your health care team.

Your Preferences for Treatment

As you've learned so far, there are several courses of treatment for endometriosis, depending largely on your symptoms and the severity of the disease. Every alternative involves some risks, inconvenience, or side effects. Your doctor needs to know your preferences and any concerns you have that might influence your treatment choices. And the physician must respect any decision you make to retain as much of your reproductive system as you choose, whether you plan to have children or not. This information will help you and your doctor design a treatment plan most likely to meet your needs. When your doctor recommends a particular treatment, ask detailed questions:

- Are there real choices?
- What are the benefits of this treatment?
- What are the risks involved?
- What are my other options?
- What should I do first?
- What are the probable outcomes of each of these options?
- What are the probable outcomes if I decide against this approach?
- How do you measure the outcome of your treatment, and for how long do you collect that information?

- If the recommended treatment is unsuccessful, what do you recommend as a subsequent course of treatment?
- Does this treatment approach temporarily mask or relieve symptoms, or does it actually remove disease?

Given the risks and benefits of the tests or treatments your doctor is recommending, consider the following questions:

- What are your treatment preferences, if any?
- What concerns or fears do you have about specific tests or treatments, if any?
- How bothersome are your symptoms? Would you prefer to live with them rather than accept the costs and risks of the test or treatment?
- Do you have the option of postponing your decision about tests or treatments?
- What lifestyle adjustments (such as diet or exercise changes) are you willing to make to manage your condition? How confident are you in your ability to make these changes?

Then ask your doctor about the things that concern you the most.

Seeking a Second Opinion

Typically, if your doctor suspects endometriosis, a laparoscopy will be recommended. Since this is the only procedure that leads to a conclusive diagnosis and provides information about the extent and severity of the disease, you could expect a second opinion at this stage to echo the first opinion. Whether to proceed with surgery is always up to you.

However, there may be situations when a second opinion is clearly advisable. Sometimes your doctor may refer you to a colleague or a specialist to confirm a diagnosis or treatment approach. You may also request another opinion for a variety of reasons, especially if you have concerns about a recommended course of treatment. Also, check with your insurance provider on its policy regarding second opinions. Some require second opinions before surgery.

The Gynecological Sourcebook suggests that a second opinion is always warranted before the following procedures:
- Hysterectomy
- Ovary removal (unless for ovarian cancer)
- D&C
- Preventive surgery

Getting Care for Related Health Problems

If you suspect that an autoimmune condition is adding to your health burdens, getting correctly diagnosed may remind you of the sometimes-difficult road that leads to an endometriosis diagnosis. Women frequently see five or six doctors before they find someone who can identify what autoimmune condition they have.

There's no one specialist to see for autoimmune disease. Various medical specialists often treat these illnesses symptom by symptom: rheumatologists for joint pain and fatigue, endocrinologists for hormone imbalances, dermatologists for rashes, and so on. As with endometriosis, if a doctor dismisses symptoms or says they are simply stress-related, seek another doctor until you find one that will travel down the road with you to identify the source of your problems.

Autoimmune Specialists

- A dermatologist treats problems of the skin, hair, and nails, including psoriasis.
- An endocrinologist treats gland and hormone problems like endometriosis, diabetes, polycystic ovarian syndrome (PCOS), and thyroid disease.
- A gastroenterologist treats problems associated with the digestive system, including Crohn's disease and ulcerative colitis.
- A hematologist treats diseases that affect the blood, including pernicious anemia and autoimmune hemolytic anemia.
- A nephrologist treats kidney problems, such as inflamed kidneys associated with lupus.
- A neurologist treats nerve problems, including multiple sclerosis and myasthenia gravis.
- A rheumatologist treats arthritis and other rheumatic diseases, which include scleroderma and systemic lupus erythematosus (lupus or SLE).

Seven Steps to Diagnosis

To help people with confusing symptoms obtain a correct diagnosis, the American Autoimmune Related Diseases Association recommends these steps:

1. Inventory your family medical history. Since current research points to a genetic component in most autoimmune diseases, learn the health histories of your close relatives, including grandparents and cousins, if possible. Share this information with your doctor, who can then form some hypotheses and order appropriate tests.

2. Keep a symptoms list. Make a list of every major symptom you've experienced in your life to present to your doctor. List the symptoms in the order of concern to you. Give a copy of the list to the nurse to be included in your records. Mention at the very start of your consultation with your doctor the symptom(s) that concerns you the most. This is often the problem to which your doctor will pay the most attention.

3. Seek referrals to good physicians. Because there is no medical specialty of "autoimmunologist," it can be difficult to determine the type of doctor you may need to see. One idea is to identify the medical specialist that deals with your major symptom and then check with a major medical center for a referral to that specialty department. A number of agencies dealing specifically with autoimmune diseases maintain referral lists.

4. Inquire about the physician's experience with autoimmune disease. Ask the physician whether he or she takes care of patients with the specific disease that has been diagnosed. Generally speaking, the more patients with a particular autoimmune disease treated by the physician, the better. Also, a specialist should be adept at managing the therapies used to treat a particular autoimmune disease.

5. Get a second, third, or fourth opinion if necessary. Because autoimmunity has just begun to be recognized as the underlying cause of some one hundred known autoimmune diseases and because symptoms can be vague, many general practice

physicians don't think to test for autoimmune diseases initially. If a doctor doesn't take your symptoms seriously, find another doctor. When trying to get a correct diagnosis, it's important to be assertive.

6. Inquire about tests. Because tests for autoimmune diseases vary, and no single test can ascertain whether a patient has an autoimmune disease, be prepared for multiple diagnostic tests. Ask: What is the purpose of this test? Are there any alternatives? Is this an outpatient or inpatient procedure? Can I anticipate any pain, discomfort, or claustrophobia; and if so, can I take medication to make me more comfortable? How much does the procedure cost, and is it covered by my health insurance? Who will get the test results, and what will they tell me about my condition? Understand that although diagnostic criteria define a disease, they are sometimes uncertain.

7. Partner with your physicians to manage your disease. Your partnership with your doctors should be active and mutual. When deciding on a treatment plan, don't be afraid to ask questions: What are the treatment options? What are the advantages and disadvantages of each? How long will the treatment last?

Treating Autoimmune Conditions

When a diagnosis has been arrived at, the primary emphasis of treating the autoimmune disease will be the correction of major biochemical deficiencies. An example would be replacing hormones that are not being produced by a particular gland, such as thyroxin in autoimmune thyroid disease or insulin in type 1 diabetes.

Second in importance is diminishing the activity of the immune system. This calls for a delicate balancing act: controlling the disorder while maintaining the body's ability to fight disease in general. The drugs most commonly used are corticosteroid drugs. Symptoms of some mild forms of rheumatic autoimmune diseases are treated with non-steroidal anti-inflammatory drugs (NSAIDs). Severe disorders may be treated with powerful immunosuppressant drugs. Such drugs, however, can damage rapidly dividing tissues, such as the bone marrow, and so are used with caution. To reduce circulating immune complexes, intra-venous immunoglobulin therapy is used in the treatment of various autoimmune diseases. Drugs that act more specifically on the immune system, for example by blocking a particular hypersensitivity reaction, are being researched.

Following the treatment plan designed by your physician is vital. If you have doubts or concerns about the treatment approach, ask questions or get a second or even a third opinion. Be sure you understand the side effects of medications and medical tests and the effect or benefit they will have on your condition.

Let your doctor know if a new symptom is occurring. Avoid the trap of worrying that your doctor will think you're whining. Physicians treating autoimmune conditions realize that symptoms are varied and may seem unrelated; your honesty in keeping the physician informed about any changes in your condition is important for appropriate treatment.

Remember, your doctor is your partner in improving your health. Be honest with your doctor, and take an active role in your treatment plan. Once you're satisfied that the plan is right for you, follow it.

Dietitians

Registered dietitians are a tremendous and often underutilized source of nutritional knowledge when it comes to dealing with chronic illnesses. People with diabetes have traditionally been the most likely to use the services of a registered dietitian to help them establish a solid eating program, because diabetes has such a direct link to nutrition and how the body utilizes food. But as I said in Chapter Eight, diet is an important issue for women with endometriosis.

Bringing a registered dietitian (look for the initials RD after someone's name) onto your health care team can save you a lot of personal research and experimentation—why reinvent the wheel when the dietitian has been trained to know these things? According to the American Dietetic Association's *Complete Food and Nutrition Guide*, an RD is "an authority on the role of food and nutrition in health. To earn the RD credential, an individual must complete at least four years of education in a nutrition or a related field from a regionally accredited college or university that's approved by the American Dietetic Association [ADA]." Graduates can specialize and often go on for advanced degrees. To use the RD credentials, dietitians must pass an extensive exam administered by the testing agency of the ADA and must complete at least seventy-five hours of continuing education every five years to stay current. The ADA is located in Chicago and is over 70,000 members strong.

You can get names of RDs in your area through the ADA's Consumer Nutrition Hotline at 800-366-1655 or on their web site at www.eatright.org. You can also get referrals through your physician, local hospital, public health department, or regional/state dietetic association.

Naturopaths

If you like the idea of actively participating in improving your overall well-being and are interested in alternative approaches to health care, adding a naturopath to your medical team is worth serious consideration. Naturopathic physicians, with their focus on a widerange of techniques to promote the healing process instead of suppressing symptoms, can also serve as primary care physicians.

Naturopathic medicine is founded on the idea that the body is its own best healer. Treatment, which is as non-invasive as possible, is directed toward identifying the root of the problem and then providing the body with natural tools so it can heal and repair itself. Many of the underlying concepts of naturopathic medicine, such as a healthy, natural diet and stress management, are now fully integrated into conventional medicine.

Naturopathic medicine is founded on seven principles:

1. First, do no harm.
2. Facilitate and enhance the natural healing capacities of the body.
3. Identify and treat the cause.
4. Treat the whole person.

5. The naturopathic physician is a teacher.

6. Prevention is the best cure.

7. Establish and maintain optimal health: physical, mental, and emotional.

In accordance with these principles, naturopathic doctors make recommendations for how you can strengthen the building blocks of good health through modifications in lifestyle, diet, and exercise. Some practitioners specialize in a particular approach, while others draw on a wide range of techniques. Common therapies include botanical medicine, homeopathy, traditional Chinese medicine (TCM), detoxification, touch therapies, shiatsu, massage, counseling, and psychotherapies.

Like traditional (allopathic) doctors, naturopaths begin the process of clinical assessment with a complete medical history, physical examinations, and laboratory tests as required. Other diagnostic techniques may also be used. For instance, a naturopath trained in TCM may use pulse diagnosis to gain information about the flow of qi and then use acupuncture to address blockages or excesses in energy flow.

Typically, the first office visit takes an hour and includes a thorough medical and lifestyle history. Diagnostic tests such as urinalysis and blood work may be scheduled to gather additional information about your health. Based on the findings, you and the doctor work together to establish a treatment plan centered on enhancing the body's immune responses. In general, treatment is directed toward cleansing therapies to reduce accumulated waste and toxins in the body or toward strengthening the body, primarily through nutrition.

Your willing participation and commitment to treatment are vital to successful work with a naturopath. If you are ready to be an active partner in the process of helping your body, mind, and spirit diminish the effects of endometriosis, a naturopath might be the perfect addition to your health care team.

Be in Control!

As you can see, your health care team is important in successfully controlling any chronic illness. You are in the driver's seat and can hire and fire members of your team. In the process, you'll form a group of people who are on your side and have the same approach to your health care as you do. It is a critical part of your success in managing endometriosis.

CHAPTER ELEVEN ∾

Your Support Network

This is the most important chapter in this book!

The symptoms of endometriosis are as individual as each woman who has this complex condition. That it is not contagious nor, in and of itself, life threatening does not lessen the fact that it is frustrating, complicated, and often very painful.

Although the symptoms of endometriosis aren't visible for the most part, they can still have a significant impact on intimate relationships and even everyday life. In fact, endometriosis not being visible can make it that much more difficult for friends and family to understand the severity of your experience.

However, endometriosis is difficult to deal with alone. Support from family, friends, and professionals is critical to the successful management of endo. Only you can decide how detailed you will get with family members and friends about your symptoms and endometriosis diagnosis. But unless it is extremely mild, endometriosis will have some effect on your family and social life.

The women interviewed for this book shared stories about being constantly sidelined from family gatherings or social events by the symptoms of endo. From heavy bleeding to pain, fatigue, and never knowing quite when your period is going to start, you name it, endometriosis got in the way of their day-to-day plans. Marybeth, who finally was diagnosed and gained control of the disease, even recalled seeing her cousin's eyes light up when she caught sight of Marybeth as the cousin walked down the aisle for her wedding; the bride later explained that she had always thought of Marybeth as the sickly family member who always either retreated to a dark bedroom at gatherings or didn't show up at all.

For something with invisible causes, endometriosis can have such a visible effect on relationships, and feeling supported can be a struggle at best. But it's important to do what you can to develop a support network.

Dealing with Pain

Pain, as you know, is one of the most significant symptoms of endometriosis for many women. Pain is such a personal thing that it is often hard for others to relate to the level of pain you may be experiencing. However, the following quote (from *The Miller-Keane Encyclopedia and Dictionary of Medicine, Nursing, and Allied Health* as quoted in *The Endometriosis Sourcebook*) may help: "Pain...is present when the person who is experiencing it says it is." It's as simple as that. If you feel pain, then you feel pain.

Women have long been subject to being considered melodramatic about the natural bodily changes that take place each month as the menstrual cycle ebbs and flows and to be considered quite frail. While men have a tradition of avoiding their health issues and being concerned only when something dramatic happens—like a heart attack—and they can no longer avoid it, women have often been told to be more stoic, that they make too much of things.

Do not fall prey to the attitude that your pain is insignificant or should simply be withstood. There are many indirect ways to deal with pain by ameliorating the symptoms of endometriosis and direct ways of dealing with the actual pain, be it a chronic headache or pain during intercourse caused by excessive vaginal dryness.

If you find someone to talk with about your pain, that's great. Support is always good. If you don't have a person in your life with whom you can share your aches and pains and know that instead of being criticized or asked to stop, you will get sympathy and relief, you still do not have to go it completely alone. However, be aware that someone who has not experienced the kind of pain you are living with is not going to be able to empathize with you and may even have a hard time sympathizing. For a while you may find a particular person a great sounding board, but if they can't empathize—i.e., they haven't been there—then their empathy is going to wane. Don't be critical of them; think of the many times that friends and family members have poured their financial, marital, relationship, child-rearing, or career woes on you. It was OK for a while, right? You were happy to provide a sympathetic ear, to be someone who was uninvolved for them to unload on. But if that was the extent of your relationship every time you were with this person, then you surely got tired of it. Either you started to avoid that person or you tuned out what they were saying; sometimes, you probably didn't believe any more that their problems could be that extensive.

It will be the same with your management of endometriosis. Don't pretend to all your friends and family that everything is fine with your health, but find outlets for some of your complaints. Perhaps someone who isn't personally involved with you can lend a sympathetic ear because he/she is either a professional in the field or an empathetic endometriosis patient herself.

I don't mean that you don't need to have that personal support network, too. There are many ways to get the overall support you need to get through the day, the week, the diagnosis, and the treatment.

In contemporary times, so much more is known about the natural functioning of the female reproductive system, from the menstrual cycle to menopause, and the things that can go wrong in the body's systems. As always, we live in the best of times and the worst of times. About some things, medical science knows just enough to make things more frustrating but not enough to do anything concrete about it. We are coming to understand many more diseases and conditions—fibromyalgia, polycystic ovarian syndrome, and Alzheimer's, to name just a few—but we still do not fully understand the root causes and therefore cannot be proactive with confidence.

If you have been diagnosed with endometriosis, now is the time to focus on managing it. Your health and well-being are in your hands. In previous chapters, you read about all the specific physical and physiological treatments available. You also need to deal with your mental and emotional health.

You Are Not a Hypochondriac

If you've had endometriosis for a long time, you may have found that you are often unable to attend family functions or your attendance is restricted or shortened by endometriosis. Again, because the symptoms of endometriosis are not visible to the people around you, you may be made to feel like a hypochondriac. At least with a broken arm you have a cast, with a cold your nose is running, and with a stomach bug you are vomiting loud enough for everyone to know that you aren't quite right! You need to find ways to deal with the fact that you know that something is wrong. Once you have a definitive diagnosis, you will probably get taken more seriously anyway—and by then, hopefully you are well down the road to reducing your symptoms!

Of course, it is easy to say that you know what is wrong, and therefore you simply need to ignore the skeptics. But that is much easier said than done. Humans are social creatures, and what people think of us and how much interaction we can have with others have a real impact on the way we feel overall.

Depression

With any chronic condition comes the possibility of depression at some point as you attempt to manage the condition. The seemingly overwhelming task of trying to control the condition itself can sap your time and energy. Depression can be more severe for women who have experienced a long period of unsuccessful attempts to get pregnant. And for women who have symptoms that make relationships difficult, the lack of a partner and the accompanying feelings can be triggers for depression as well.

First, accept that depression is a very real thing. If you have some or all of these classic signs:

- Feeling down for more than a couple days in a row,
- Avoiding having a social life and preferring to stay at home by yourself,
- Crying episodes that don't have evident provocation, and
- Being overly critical of yourself,

don't hesitate to pick up the phone and make an appointment with your doctor. Be frank with her or him about your feelings, and get a referral to a therapist or counselor who can help you work through these emotional ups and downs.

Your doctor will also want to work with you on other possible causes of your depression. It may not be a reaction to endometriosis itself, but perhaps to the medication you are on to treat your symptoms.

If you feel like your family or even the world would be better off without you around, please do not ignore those feelings. See a doctor or a professional counselor immediately. Suicidal feelings must be taken seriously. The symptoms and treatments for endometriosis can be overwhelming, and there are people who can help.

Sometimes, diagnosis and the start of a treatment plan can in itself help raise your spirits. Being diagnosed with any chronic condition is not a happy occasion, but often a diagnosis can bring with it the relief of having a name for your symptoms and a direction to take to alleviate pain.

Be kind to yourself. Now that you have a diagnosis and are taking care of your physical health, don't forget your mental and emotional health as well.

Pick-Me-Ups

Most women, thankfully, do not experience clinical depression as the result of endometriosis. However, the complexity of the condition and your attempts to manage it can sometimes make you feel overwhelmed. Top that off with a job, relationship, and family, and anyone would feel like she had quite a bit on her plate.

Be sure to treat yourself to stress relievers and other activities that make you feel better. Exercise is hard to consider when you are in pain, but exercise also offers the benefits of natural stress-relieving endorphin release, which can help improve your feelings. Don't think that you have to run a marathon to get exercise! Start small. Walk around the block. The key with exercise as a mood elevator is that the exercise is regular (at least three days a week) and that each exercise period lasts for thirty minutes or more. Find a lovely public garden near your home or work to stroll through every couple of days. If you don't have your own, borrow the neighbor's dog to walk to the park, sit on a bench, and toss a ball for it. Animals have a way of putting a smile on almost everyone's face!

Relationship Issues

Some women interviewed for this book put having an intimate relationship on hold while they tried to figure out what was going on with their bodies. Other women discovered their endometriosis in the midst of attempting to get pregnant while in a committed relationship. Whatever the case with you, endo can take a toll on relationships.

It is essential that your partner, if you have one, be supportive of your condition and the effect it has on your day-to-day life. But people who do not have endometriosis cannot know exactly what you are dealing with—it is up to you to help your partner understand what you are going through so that your partner can support you when you need it the most.

Support to you may be simply taking the trash out, fixing a nice dinner, or perhaps skipping that night out with co-workers to come home and help you get through the evening. One of the main advantages of having a partner is that kind of support, so let your partner know what would help you out today. A partner is not a mind reader; if you just tell him or her exactly what could make your day go a little more smoothly, he or she is usually more than willing to do it.

One of the most critical areas of a relationship has to do with sex. Many women who have endometriosis suffer from pain with intercourse. This is an area where communication with your partner is critical. Certain positions can be less painful, or sometimes activities other than vaginal intercourse may be desirable. Dealing with endo can be an opportunity for a couple to talk freely about their sexual relationship and even improve it. In fact, the educational process of discussing this sensitive issue with your partner may be helpful in the overall success of your relationship.

Another thing that may help your partner understand more of what you are going through is to have the partner accompany you to an appointment with your doctor. We all know what it's like trying to relate secondhand what someone said to us, trying to remember the details and the best way to phrase things after listening intently to a whole appointment's worth of information. Have your partner come along and let him or her hear straight from the doctor what he needs to know to understand your bad days and your need for support. You will also want him to be knowledge-able enough about your condition to help you make crucial medical decisions, such as whether to take particular medications given their potential side effects or, if your endo is severe, whether to have a hysterectomy.

If your partner is unwilling to be as involved as you would like, you need to be up front with him about your needs. Since endometriosis that does not have a known cure, you will be managing it for a long time and, therefore, so will he! Men often don't like to hear all the gory details about medical-related topics, so perhaps you need to get the real scoop from him about how detailed you can be in discussions with him. Above all, the simple fact of the matter is that your spouse or significant other is a key partner in your health and you need to be able to rely on him (or her, if you are in an alternative relationship) for support. The onus is on you to make sure that happens.

Sex and the Woman With Endometriosis

When you are in pain, it's probably safe to say that sex isn't at the top of your list of eagerly anticipated activities. And many women with endometriosis describe sexual intercourse as extremely physically painful.

As you work with your doctor on your diagnosis and treatment, of course you're working toward having a normal level of activity in all aspects of your life, including sex. In the meantime, you probably want to find ways to satisfy your sexual desires without having to be in pain. Perhaps you need to consider means of sexual relations other than intercourse until you get the endometriosis under control and reduce your pain during intercourse. Perhaps you don't need to avoid intercourse completely. You can simply figure out what days of the month or even times of the day you feel your best and set aside some of that time for intimacy with your partner.

You may want to try doing some things before intimacy that relax you, such as taking a warm bath or hot shower or learning to give each other relaxing massages.

It may seem hard to be innovative about your sex life when you are trying to manage endometriosis, but don't ignore it. Remember to communicate—a good relationship is worth it!

Your Doctor

As discussed in Chapter Ten, your primary care physician is a critical member of your support network, as are all the members of your health team, from your dietitian to your obstetrician/gynecologist

(OB/GYN) to your homeopath to your personal trainer. Although they differ from family and friends by the sheer fact that they get paid for the services they provide you, there is still a reason these professionals chose what are known as the "helping professions." They get great satisfaction from helping people.

If you do not feel that your doctor or another member of your health care team is providing you with the support that can be reasonably expected, you should definitely shop around for someone new. Just be sure you understand from the beginning what reasonable expectations are. You can't expect your primary care physician to drop everything and talk with you every time you call, whether it's five times a day or once a week. However, if you have a serious problem or question, you should be able to expect a call back within twenty-four hours (anything more serious than that warrants an urgent care/emergency room visit or a prompt office appointment).

Sometimes you'll find that the personal style of one of the members of your medical team just doesn't mesh with yours. This is an important part of support, too. You need to feel comfortable with the people who are caring for you. Find someone else to fill that role; there are other dietitians, personal trainers, and even doctors who may be a better match. If you don't feel comfortable with the people who are caring for you, you won't be comfortable telling them what they need to know to give you the best care.

Your Family

Your next line of support after your partner is probably your family. If you live near your immediate family, they will probably be very aware of the effects of endometriosis on your life. They may also remember your teenage years, when the days around your menstrual cycle incapacitated you so much that you couldn't attend family functions, get out of bed, go to school, or even eat dinner.

Again, how open you are with your family is entirely up to you. If you are not geographically close, you can probably get away with not telling them much. But if your family members are supportive as a rule, whether close by or not, they can be a key element in your support network that you should be sure to lean on if you need to.

If a sister lives nearby, perhaps she would be a good choice to come to an occasional doctor's appointment with you to help you sort through the maze of information. If you're not in an intimate relationship, now may be the time to ask your mom to help you with the details of managing endometriosis. Of course, it all depends on your family relationships, but if they are strong, be sure to utilize them.

Friends

Like family, good friends are often just waiting to be asked to help. Your closest friends have probably already figured out that something is going on, especially when you cancel plans at the last minute or don't feel like joining the group on a Saturday night out. Women friends are some of the most special relationships, and now is the time to let your friends help you.

Because endometriosis is characterized by a lot of pain and discomfort, you need to be careful not to complain all the time. But good friends know that sometimes a little complaining to each other is just what friends are for.

If you are up-front about how you are feeling, maybe the group would sometimes all agree to enjoy a nice quiet Saturday evening at your place with delivered pizza and a rented movie—you don't have to go anywhere, you can avoid feeling left home alone on a Saturday night, and, depending on how close your friends are, you could probably watch the movie in your pajamas!

Work Life

If you have a job or are trying hard to establish a strong career in any field, the side effects of endometriosis can be devastating. Most of the women interviewed for this book had very understanding and accommodating employers and co-workers. But if you want to be on the fast track or are in a career that requires a lot of travel or requires your attendance at many functions, it may be challenging to manage endometriosis while balancing your career.

First, if your employer is being less than cooperative, find out what your employment rights are. Document any instances where you are unjustly treated. And if you are in a company big enough to have one, talk with the human rights department. While your employer expects you to be able to do the job you were hired for, you also have the right not to be discriminated against for medical reasons.

That said, don't expect your employer to always do the accommodating. On bad days, perhaps you can do some work at home for a few hours when you feel up to it—and in your pajamas propped up in bed. Perhaps on days when your flow is so excessive that you just can't be in the office, you could make phone calls from home or attend meetings via conference call. Let your employer see that you are trying hard to work around your medical issues if at all possible. Making an effort is sometimes all it takes to get more support than you might otherwise. This will also help your co-workers to be more supportive; if you are sensitive to the fact that they probably have to shoulder some of the excess work when you are out, they may be very helpful in assisting you to work around those down days.

Support Groups

Online Chat Rooms and Discussion Groups

Many women report getting a lot out of going online and joining some chat rooms and discussion groups specific to endometriosis. Almost every illness from cancer to headaches has an online support group.

Look first on the larger endometriosis-specific web sites for chat room and discussion group sites. You might also find them on the larger general medical web sites as well, such as the Mayo Clinic and the National Institutes of Health.

If you want some support and ideas about a specific endometriosis symptom, search for that symptom on the Internet and look for sites that have ongoing support groups for that symptom. For instance, you may be interested in finding support specifically for pain management or sex-related issues, not just endometriosis in general.

Listen in for a while (also called "lurking" when you listen in on a chat room but don't join in) and see what people are talking about. Figure out what the attitude of the group is. Some groups are pretty straightforward and not interested in providing moral support as much as providing solid information. It may be helpful for you to hear the information, but it may not be the best group for emotional support. If you are sensitive, you don't want to ask a question and be chastised for bringing up a topic the group (or, usually, a couple very active members) don't want to talk about. Just with like any group of people discussing any topic, you will want to be comfortable with the atmosphere of the group.

When you pick a group to become active with, learn the rules of the group so you don't risk a sharp response from an innocent but inappropriate question. Keep in mind that one of the good things about online chatting is that you can leave the group at any time never to return, and you won't see one of the members in the grocery store (or if you do, neither of you will know it) and have to explain why you left the group.

Lastly, remember that not all of the information you receive in a chat room or discussion group (or anywhere online for that matter) is necessarily accurate. Chat room members can forget the name of the drug they are taking or call it something else; they can exaggerate the benefits of a treatment, not fully understand the treatment they are undergoing, or not understand the details of their specific diagnosis. That doesn't make support groups less valuable. Just don't be surprised if you demand that you be put on Lupron because a chat room member was completely cured of endo by taking Lupron for a week, and your doctor says no! If something seems valid and you want to research it and discuss it with your doctor, who will research it too, that's completely appropriate—doctors can't know everything about every disease and drug out there. However, they also will not prescribe potent medication on the whim of a chat room discussion.

Also be sure to follow all the usual safety guidelines when it comes to chatting on support group sites and other discussion groups. Never give out your address or even phone number to the general group; if you establish a personal e-mail relationship with one individual with whom you end up talking on the phone, that's great, but you don't need to broadcast your personal information to do that.

If you search for "support groups" on the Internet, then narrow your search to "endometriosis," you will find plenty of options. Some require membership, others don't, but they are all in abundance. Here are a few to get you started:

- *Yahoo!Groups* at *http://groups.yahoo.com* has an endometriosis group, as does GoogleGroups at *http://groups.google.com.* Some topics include "endometriosis and kidneys and bladder," "Anyone else here on Depo-Provera?", and "Questions about Lupron."

- The site *www.endowisdom.com* has a whole list of support groups, including a breakdown by state. The group under St. Augustine, Florida, has a doctor as a sponsor; as with any online information, this is the kind of credibility to look for.

- The site *www.obgyn.net* was designed predominately for doctors but is now expanding into dissemination of information to the public also. This site now has the Endometriosis Zone (*www.endozone.org*), which can be a resource for patients and has articles and interviews on current treatment of endometriosis.

- My own web site, Center for Women's Care & Reproductive Surgery *(www.thomasllyons.com* or *www.endocenter.com*), has both educational articles and an interactive site for questions about this and other related topics and gynecologic problems.

- The Endometriosis Research Center, which claims to "bridge the gap between science and support," has a Web site (*www.endocenter.org*) with support groups.

- The site *www.supportpath.com* lists online support groups in dozens of topics within the categories of relationships, personal, and health-related, including endometriosis. The site also includes good links to other sites and a nice list of events, although the events were out of date the day I visited the site.

- The *www.psychcentral.com* site is sponsored by Dr. John Grohol, author of the book *The Insider's Guide to Mental Health Resources Online.* The site includes live chats and book reviews, plus some humor and essays along with the doctor's personal blog. The focus is on mental health, but the topics are ones that anyone dealing with a chronic illness may be facing.

- MSN has a support network on WebMD located at *http://content.health.msn.com.* And you can create your own online support group through the MSN Support Groups page at *http://groups.msn.com.*

This is just a short list of what you may find when you run a search on the words "support groups" on the Internet. In this information and technology age you don't have to be alone, no matter where you are or how remote you are from your circle of family and friends.

In-Person Support Groups

If you would like to find a support group in your area to attend in-person meetings, ask about support groups at your doctor's office or call the local hospital. If there isn't one specific to endometriosis, perhaps the local hospital would appreciate your help in organizing one through the hospital's community education program.

There really is nothing more comforting than hearing stories from other people who have been and are going through the same thing you are. And to meet them in person and have an ongoing network of support to see you through the tough times and cheer you through the better times is important in dealing with a chronic illness.

Many hospitals are seeing the advantage of this kind of support and are happy to provide a place for such a group to meet. Much of the pioneering of this kind of support has been done by people facing life-threatening illnesses such as cancer, but any chronic illness is a prime candidate for a hospital-sponsored support group.

Some groups are more formal with speakers and guests, others are simply a group of people with the same condition sharing information. If your local hospital or the one that your doctor is part of does not have an endometriosis support group and you don't want to help start one, check the next town over or other places in the greater geographic area. It really is worth the effort.

PERSONAL STORIES

Some women with endometriosis told their stories in some of the chapters in this book. All of these women talked about what kind of support network they've had as they have worked to find a way to manage endometriosis. Here are the support aspects of a couple of their stories.

Kim

Kim's support network is strong. She is not married and moved back to her hometown after divorcing her husband several years ago. As a teacher, she has found her co-workers, boss, and even her students to be very understanding about the times during the month when endometriosis plays a large part in what she can and can't do. Her boss has made it clear to her that family and health come first—without these two things, you cannot be a good employee.

Kim has found it most difficult to cope with the number of people around her who are having children. Many women at work are or have been pregnant. Her sister is pregnant. Kim has wanted nothing more desperately in her life than to have children. She was unable to get pregnant when she was with her husband; her doctor did not think it was impossible for her to get pregnant, so she thought maybe her husband was the one with a fertility problem. But he has since remarried and had children with his second wife.

Now that Kim has had recent surgery for endometriosis, her doctor has told her it is a prime time for her to get pregnant. However, she is not married, does not have a partner, and does not see a serious relationship in her near future. She has considered artificial insemination through a sperm bank and other options for pregnancy. Kim has worried about how her parents would take this approach, so she talked openly with them about this idea. As they have been throughout her health ordeal, Kim's parents made it clear to her that they were supportive of whatever decision she made.

Despite all of this great support, Kim wishes that she knew someone who had more of a direct idea of all she is going through. She has decided it is probably time to join some sort of support group, either online or via the local hospital.

Carrie

Both Carrie's family and friends have provided her with great support. She also felt that her medical professionals were very supportive and always took her complaints seriously. In fact, she had almost never complained to her doctor over the years, so when she went to her OB/GYN with her endometriosis symptoms and complained of severe pain, her doctor took her very seriously.

However, Carrie admits, unless someone has been through the entire ordeal herself, it is virtually impossible to empathize with what she was going through. There is no way to understand the actual pain and other complications brought about by endometriosis unless you feel them yourself.

Carrie never felt alone though, however. She did check in with chat rooms and discussion groups. Although she never posted her own experiences, asked questions, or participated in the online support groups that she listened in on, she spent a lot of time reading message boards dedicated to endometriosis. By reading everyone else's experiences, she could be assured that she was not the only one in the world going through this ordeal—that she was not alone.

Carrie feels that it is important for every woman with endometriosis to find some way to connect with other women who have endo. If you don't know anyone personally, she feels strongly that you should do whatever it takes—check out online groups, ask your doctor, go to support groups in your medical community—to find other women to network with, not just for the information and knowledge you may gain about the disease, but for the sheer comfort of knowing that you are not alone.

GLOSSARY ∿

adenomyosis: endometriosis

adhesions: scar tissues that stretch between two surfaces, connecting areas that would not normally meet

allergen: a substance that induces allergy

anaphylaxic reaction: a group of symptoms that represent a sometimes overwhelming and dangerous allergic reaction due to extreme hypersensitivity to a drug.

atopic: not in the usual place

autoimmune disorders: disorders where the body's antibodies attacks its own body tissue

BCPs: birth control pills

biofeedback therapy: making unconscious or involuntary bodily processes (heartbeat or brainwaves) perceptible to the senses (as by use of an oscilloscope) in order to manipulate them by conscious mental control

candidas: an infection caused by a common yeast-like fungus, candida albicans.

cecum: a part of the digestive system where the large intestine begins

corpus luteum: The follicle after it is empty of an egg

cul–de–sac: posterior area of the pelvic cavity

diverticular disease: inflammation of a pocket that is diverting off froma hollow organ such as the intestine

dysmenorrhea: painful menstruation

dyschezia: painful bowel movements

dyspareunia: difficult or painful intercourse

ectopic pregnancy: a potentially life-threatening condition in which the fertilized egg implants and begins to develop outside the uterus, most often in the fallopian tubes

endorphins: proteins occurring naturally in the brain that have pain relieving properties

estradiol: one of the three types of estrogen produced by the body

estriol: one of the three types of estrogen produced by the body

estrone: one of the three types of estrogen produced by the body

excisional surgery: removal of disease using a cutting instrument

extirpation: to cut out by surgery

fibrin: a white insoluble fibrous protein capable of being solubilized by certain enzymes

fibromyalgia: an autoimmune syndrome characterized by pain and difficulty moving.

FSH: Follicle Stimulating Hormone, the hormone that stimulates the egg follicle in the ovary to ovulate

gamete intrafallopian transfer (GIFT): is a technique where a surgeon removes ripe eggs from the ovaries and immediately places them in the fallopian tubes along with sperm.

GnRH: Gonadotrophin Releasing Hormone, which stimulates the production of FSH at the appropriate time

histamine: a substance that is the main culprit of allergic reactions

hysterosalpingogram: a test which determines whether the uterus is a normal shape and the fallopian tubes are open

IBS: Irritable Bowel Syndrome

intrauterine insemination (IUI): a doctor injects concentrated sperm into the uterus

kallikreins: a hypotensive proteinase that liberates kinins from blood plasma proteins and is used therapeutically for vasodilation

laparoscopy: surgery by means of a camera and instruments inserted through a small incision, in the case of endometriosis, in the abdominal wall

LH: Luteinizing Hormone, which stimulates the manufacture of testosterone

libido: the desire for sexual gratification

menorrhagia: heavy menstrual bleeding

methylcellulose barrier: used to surfaces from rubbing together post-surgery and have proven to be very effective in reducing post-surgical adhesion formation

moxibusiton: medical use of a "moxa" or substance used as a counterirritant

myofascial: pertaining to the surface area of the muscles

NSAIDs: Non Steroidal Anti Inflammatory Drugs

nociceptors: pain sensing organs

oopharectomy: removal of the ovaries

peptides: any of a class of amides that are derived from two or more amino acids

pericardium: the sac around the heart

peritoneum: thin membrane protecting pelvic organs and abdominal cavity

postcoital test: a test that determines whether sperm can survive the trip to meet the egg

progestogenic drugs: any of several progestational steroids (as progesterone)

prostaglandins: any of various oxygenated unsaturated cyclic fatty acids of animals that perform a variety of hormonelike actions (as in controlling blood pressure or smooth muscle contraction)

reproductive endocrinologist: physicians who received formal obstetrics and gynecology subspecialty training in the field of hormonal regulation of reproduction and the treatment of infertility

rhinitis: hay fever

rolfing: deep tissue body work

SHBG: Sex-hormone Binding Globulin

synovia: a transparent viscid lubricating fluid found in joints

systemic: affecting the body in general

TCM: Traditional Chinese Medicine

vasoconstrictive: constricting blood vessels

zygote intrafallopian tranfer (ZIFT): a surgeon retrieves eggs which are then combined with sperm in a dish. The resulting zygotes are then placed in the fallopian tubes, where they can travel on their own into the uterus, with increased odds of pregnancy.

RESOURCES ∿

Alternatives for Women with Endometriosis: A Guide by Women for Women. Ruth Carol, ed. 1994. Third Side Press, Chicago, IL.

Endometrium & Endometriosis. Diamond M. & Osteen K, eds. 1997. Blackwell Science, Malden, MA.

Surgical Management of Endometriosis. Redwine D., ed. 2003. Martin Dunitz Publishers, London, UK.

The American Dietetic Association's Complete Food & Nutrition Guide. 2002. Roberta Duyff Wiley, Hoboken, NJ.

Earl Mindell's Supplement Bible. Earl Mindell. 1998. Fireside, New York, NY.

The Encyclopedia and Dictionary of Medicine, Nursing, and Allied Health, 5th Edition. 1992. W. B. Saunders Co, Philadelphia, Pa.

Encyclopedia of Healing Therapies. Anne Woodham & Dr. David Peters. 1997. Dorling Kindersley Ltd., London, UK.

Encyclopedia of Natural Medicine. Michael Murray, N.D. and Pizzorno, Joseph, N.D. 2nd Revised Ed. 1998. Prima Publishing, Rocklin, CA.

Endometriosis: A Natural Approach. Jo Mears. 1998. Ulysses Press, Berkeley, CA.

Endometriosis Sourcebook. Mary Lou Ballweg and the Endometriosis Association. 1995. Contemporary Books, Chicago, IL.

The Gynecological Sourcebook. M. Sara Rosenthal. Updated edition, 1997. Lowell House, Los Angeles, CA.

Learn to Sleep Well. Chris Idzikowski. 2000. Chronicle Books, San Francisco, CA.

Natural Treatment of Fibroid Tumors and Endometriosis. Susan M. Lark, M.D. 1996. Keats Publishing, New Canaan, CT.

The Nutritional Health Handbook for Women. Marily Glenville, PhD. 2001. Piatkus, London, England.

Our Bodies, Ourselves for the New Century. The Boston Women's Health Collective. 1998.

Simon & Schuster, New York, NY.

Prescription for Nutritional Healing. James F. Balch, M.D. & Phyllis A. Balch, C.N.C. 2nd edition, 1997. Avery Publishing Group, Avery Park, NY.

What to Do When the Doctor Says It's PCOS. Milton Hammerly M.D. and Cheryl Kimball. 2003. Fair Winds Press, Gloucester, MA.

A Woman's Guide to Staying Healthy Through Her 30s. Theresa Francis-Cheung. 2002. Adams Media, Avon, MA.

The Yeast Connection. William G. Crook, M.D. 3rd edition, 1986. Vintage Books, New York, NY.

WEB SITES ∾

http://altmed.od.nih.gov: The National Center for Complementary and
Alternative Medicine

http://hcgresources.com/docs.html: Endometriosis Awareness and Information

http://womenshealth.about.com: What You Need to Know About Women's Health

www.abchomeopathy.com/c.php/endometriosis: ABC Homeopathy

www.acupuncture.com to locate a licensed practitioner in the states that license
the profession

www.aarda.org/women.html American Autoimmune Related Diseases Association

www.acupuncturetoday.com: site for *Acupuncture Today* magazine

www.all-natural.com: Natural Health and Longevity Resource Center

www.asrm.org: American Society for Reproductive Medicine

www.bidmc.harvard.edu/obgyn/problems_endo.asp: Beth Israel Deaconess
Medical Center

www.centerforendo.com/news/fertility/fertility.htm: Center for Endometriosis Care

www.clearpassage.com: Clear Passage Therapies, treatment for female infertility,
adhesions, and chronic pain

www.cnn.com/2000/HEALTH/07/04/autoimmune.disease.wmd: CNN Health

www.conceivingconcepts.com: Infertility information, products, and services

www.docrockfish.com/endometriosis.html: Rockfish Chiropractic, Reaford, NC,
natural recommendations for endometriosis

www.drlark.com: Dr. Susan Lark's website

www.eatright.com The American Dietetic Association

www.endoangels.com: EndoAngels online support group

www.endocenter.org: Nonprofit organization providing education and
support services

www.EndometriosisAssn.org: Support and services for endometriosis patients

www.endometriosis.org

www.endosupp.com: Promotes awareness, offers support, links,

    doctor recommendations

www.fertilitext.org: Fertilitext: A Family Building Network

www.gsdl.com: Allergy blood test info

www.hcgresources.com/articles.htm: Freelance articles on health education topics

www.healthlinks.net: health care directory

www.healthwell.com: natural health

www.holistic-online.com: homeopathic and herbal medicine

www.immuneweb.org: Support and information network for immune-system ailments

www.inciid.org: International Council on Infertility Information Dissemination

www.itmonline.org/journal/arts/endometriosis.htm: Article on Chinese

    herbal research

www.ivf.com: Information on IVF, endometriosis, and pelvic pain

www.jenniferlewis.com: Personal account of woman with endometriosis

www.naturopathy-anp.com: Association of Naturopathic Practitioners

www.obgyn.net: Comprehensive resources for women and health professionals

www.prevention.com: Site of *Prevention* magazine

www.pulsemed.org: Online alternative medicine magazine

www.sensiblehealth.com: Conquering Chronic Health Problems without

    Drugs or Surgery

www.susunweed.com: Susun Weed, herbalist and author, website on natural

    alternatives for women with health concerns

www.vmmc.org: Virginia Mason Medical Center in Seattle

www.webmd.com: Interactive site with news, library, dictionary

www.webwomb.com: Fertility site

www.wordplay.org: find endometriosis stories from *Endo Magazine.*

INDEX ᘓ

autoimmune system and, 122

endometriosis symptoms and, 49–52

inflammatory bowel disease, 106

irritable bowel syndrome, 80,
105–106, 128

statistics about, 33

breast-feeding, 200

C

CA 125 blood test, 83

caffeine, avoiding, 191

calcarea carb, 162

cancer, 18, 118

candida albicans, 122, 134

relief from, 156, 161–163

candidiasis, 52–53, 124–125. See also
candida albicans

carbohydrates, 168

Carlston, Dr. Michael, 155

CenterWatch, 29

cervical mucus, 195, 204

chamomile, 154

Chasteberry tree, 154, 209

chat rooms, online, 250–253

Chinese medicine, see traditional
Chinese medicine (TCM)

chiropractic, 150–151

cholesterol, 169

chronic fatigue syndrome, 80, 117,
125–126

clinical trials, 27–33, 64

complementary and alternative
medicine, 24, 141–147, 159–160,
164–165

advantages of, 143–144

biofeedback therapy, 149–150

chiropractic, 150–151

fertility and, 208–212

flower remedies, 151–152

herbal medicine, 153–155

holistic therapy, 69–72

homeopathy, 155–156, 161–163, 210

naturopathy, 156–157, 234–236

nutrition, 233–234

rolfing, 157

shiatsu, 157–158

sleep quality and, 163–164

working with therapist, 145–147

yoga, 158–159, 184

see also acupuncture; nutrition;
traditional Chinese medicine

congenital theory of endometriosis, 15

constipation, see bowel irritations

co-workers, support from, 249–250

Crook, Dr. William, 161

cul-de-sac, 54, 84

cupping, 148

cysts, 46–47, 83

D

dairy foods, avoiding, 190

Danazol, 65–66, 67, 99

Depo-Provera, 64, 65

depression, 57, 241–243

diagnosis, of autoimmune diseases,
229–231

diagnosis, of endometriosis, 18–20

research about, 27–28

surgical, 42, 81–82

diarrhea, see bowel irritations

diet, see nutrition

diethylstilbestrol (DES), 16

dietitians, 171–172, 233–234

dioxins, 16, 134–136, 189

discussion groups, online, 250–253

doctors

alternative therapy and, 142, 146

clinical trials and, 31, 33

ABOUT THE AUTHOR ∽

THOMAS L. LYONS, M.D., F.A.C.O.G.

As Medical Director of the Center for Women's Care and Reproductive Surgery in Atlanta, Dr. Lyons is on staff at the Advanced Surgery Center of Georgia, Northside Cherokee Hospital, St. Joseph's Hospital, Dunwoody Medical Center, and HealthSouth Surgery Center (Medical Director) in Atlanta. He is a Clinical Assistant Professor at Emory University Medical School and an Adjunct Assistant Professor at the University of Georgia. He has participated in numerous academic and clinical studies and authored more than 100 scholarly publications, including several chapters on endometriosis.

A graduate of the University of Georgia with an AB in Psychology and a Masters degree in Clinical and Biopsychology, Dr. Lyons earned his medical degree at the University of Colorado and financed his medical education playing football with the Denver Broncos. He completed his residency program at Colorado, 1977-1981. He was among six former scholar-athletes honored as a recipient of the NCAA Silver Anniversary Award in 1996, for those who have distinguished themselves in their careers 25 years after graduation.

Dr. Lyons is devoted to gynecologic endoscopy, pelvic reconstructive surgery and infertility. He is dedicated to the development and teaching of minimally-invasive, patient-friendly procedures to physicians worldwide. His approach to endometriosis is surgical excision of the disease, a proven treatment which removes disease below its roots rather than merely lasering it off the surface. He has demonstrated his leading edge surgical techniques for endometriosis excision on several continents.

Currently he is involved in two new studies on prevention of adhesions (scar tissue) which may result from endometriosis or prior surgery. Among his peers he is a recognized leader in exploring causes and prevention of pelvic pain, including Adhesion Related Disorder and adhesive disease.

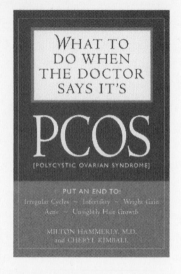